RESPIRATORY LEADERSHIP ESSENTIALS

BUILDING A CULTURE OF EXCELLENCE IN CARE

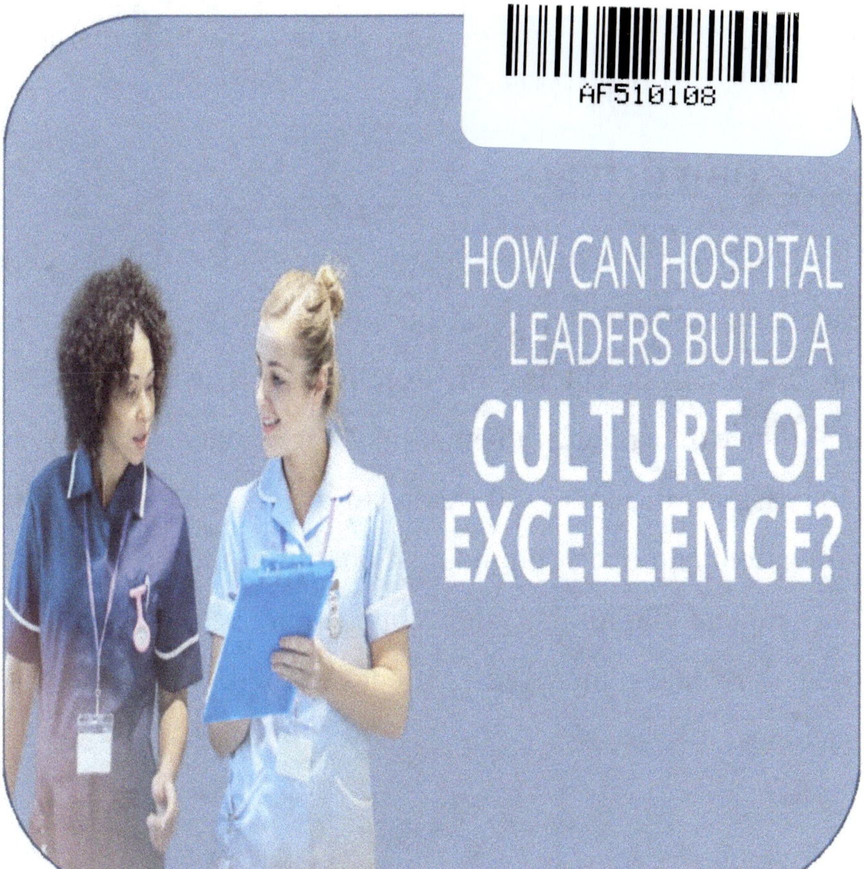

BOOK OVERVIEW

This book empowers respiratory therapy leaders to elevate clinical teams through visionary, compassionate, and accountable leadership. It explores the shift from clinician to leader, emphasizing trust, motivation, and psychological safety. Core leadership principles like emotional intelligence, ethics, and professionalism are deeply examined. By cultivating a culture of excellence, leaders can shape resilient teams and a lasting legacy in respiratory care.

BOOK OBJECTIVES

This book aims to equip respiratory care leaders with essential leadership skills, focusing on building high-performing teams and fostering a culture of excellence. It emphasizes the importance of leading with emotional intelligence, integrity, and compassion. Leaders will learn to promote accountability, motivation, and open communication within their departments. The content highlights the connection between effective leadership and improved patient-centered, evidence-based outcomes.

TABLE OF CONTENTS

INTRODUCTION

Respiratory care is a field grounded in precision, compassion, and critical thinking. Every breath a patient takes is the result of countless decisions made by professionals who understand not only the science of pulmonary health but the heart of human care. As respiratory therapists rise to meet increasingly complex clinical demands, there is a growing need for leaders who can guide, inspire, and shape the future of this vital profession. This book was born from that need.

Leadership in Respiratory Care: Excellence in Action is more than a guide, it's a call to lead with purpose. Whether you're a bedside therapist stepping into your first supervisory role, a clinical manager navigating departmental change, or a seasoned director shaping policy and practice, this book is your roadmap to becoming a confident, compassionate, and competent leader.

Leadership in healthcare doesn't come with a single definition, it's multifaceted, deeply human, and constantly evolving. In respiratory care, leadership means being the calm in the chaos of a code. It means mentoring the next generation, advocating for your patients, improving clinical outcomes, and making strategic decisions that impact lives. It means embodying excellence clinically, ethically, and relationally.

Each module combines practical tools with real-world insights, case studies, and reflection prompts to help you apply what you learn in your day-to-day practice. Whether you're managing a team, guiding a department, or preparing to lead the future of the profession, this book equips you with the mindset, skills, and strategies to lead with clarity, courage, and compassion.

Now more than ever, respiratory therapists are being recognized as essential leaders in patient care. The world needs your voice, your vision, and your commitment to excellence.

So take a deep breath.

You're not just here to respond. You're here to lead.

MODULE ONE

THE EVOLVING ROLE OF THE RESPIRATORY LEADER

THE SHIFT FROM CLINICIAN TO LEADER

Respiratory therapy is a profession grounded in skill, science, and swift clinical decision-making. For many respiratory therapists (RTs), the journey begins with mastering bedside care responding to rapid codes, managing ventilators, assessing oxygenation, and providing life-sustaining interventions. But as the healthcare landscape evolves, so too does the role of the respiratory professional. Increasingly, RTs are being called to lead: to drive team performance, shape clinical policy, and inspire a culture of excellence.

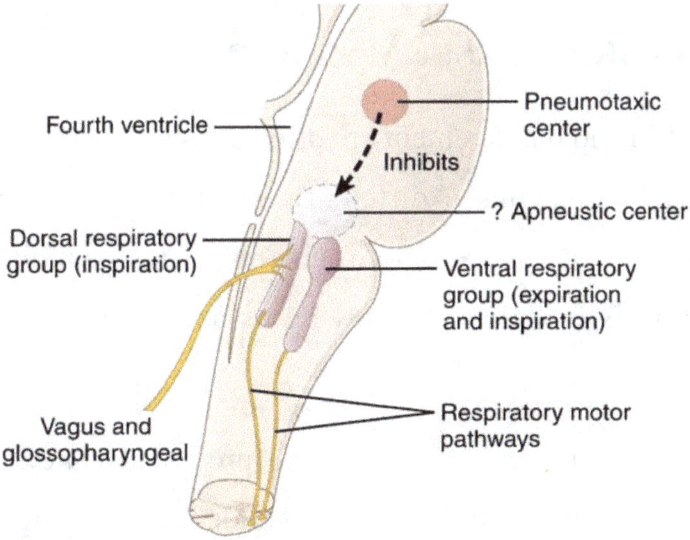

The shift from clinician to leader is not merely a change in job title, it is a transformation in mindset, responsibility, and scope. This transition often occurs subtly, beginning when a seasoned RT becomes a preceptor, then a supervisor, and eventually a department leader. Yet, each stage demands a recalibration of priorities. Where once the primary focus was direct patient care, now the emphasis expands to strategic thinking, people management, resource allocation, and fostering a high-functioning team culture.

Leaders in respiratory care must learn to balance clinical excellence with administrative effectiveness. They must advocate for their team while aligning with institutional goals. They must shift from doing to enabling from being the most skilled at the bedside to creating an environment where every team member can thrive.

LEADERSHIP VERSUS MANAGEMENT

Leadership and management are often used interchangeably, but they are fundamentally different disciplines. While both are critical in healthcare environments, understanding their distinction is essential to evolving as an effective respiratory leader.

Management focuses on systems, processes, and order. It includes scheduling staff, managing budgets, enforcing policies, and ensuring compliance. Managers aim for stability, making sure the day-to-day operations of a respiratory department run smoothly and efficiently.

Leadership, by contrast, is about vision, people, and change. Leaders inspire, influence, and create direction. They cultivate team culture, empower individuals, and promote professional growth. While managers do things right, leaders do the right things.

In an ideal department, respiratory leaders embody both roles—bringing the discipline of management together with the inspiration of leadership. But developing leadership skills requires intentional effort. It means moving beyond comfort zones, confronting difficult conversations, and taking accountability not only for clinical outcomes but also for the morale and motivation of the team.

KEY TRAITS OF SUCCESSFUL RESPIRATORY LEADERS

The most impactful leaders in respiratory care share a common set of traits. These are not innate characteristics but learned behaviors that develop through reflection, mentorship, and experience. Let's explore the key traits that define successful respiratory leaders and how they show up in practice.

1. Emotional Intelligence

At the heart of leadership lies emotional intelligence (EI)—the ability to perceive, understand, and regulate one's own emotions and respond empathetically to others. EI is especially crucial in high-stress environments like respiratory therapy, where clinicians frequently encounter life-or-death situations.

A respiratory leader with high EI can remain calm under pressure, de-escalate team tensions, and deliver feedback in a way that motivates rather than demoralizes. They recognize when a team member is struggling and offer support without judgment. They are self-aware, capable of managing their own stress to prevent it from impacting team dynamics.

2. Vision and Strategic Thinking

Great leaders have a clear vision of where their department is headed—and they know how to communicate that vision effectively. They think beyond the next shift or staff meeting. They see how their team fits into the broader goals of the hospital or health system.

Strategic thinking allows respiratory leaders to anticipate future needs, identify growth opportunities, and advocate for resources. For example, a leader might foresee the need for additional training in non-invasive ventilation and proactively develop a workshop to upskill the team.

3.Effective Communication

Whether speaking to a therapist one-on-one or presenting to hospital executives, communication is a core competency. Successful respiratory leaders are active listeners and persuasive speakers. They communicate with clarity, compassion, and confidence.

Strong communication skills are essential when conveying department goals, giving constructive feedback, and managing conflict. They also enhance interdisciplinary collaboration—ensuring that respiratory therapy is respected and integrated within broader care teams.

4. Integrity and Accountability

Trust is the currency of leadership. Respiratory leaders must operate with integrity—keeping their word, owning their mistakes, and setting a moral example. Integrity builds credibility and reinforces psychological safety among team members.

Accountability is closely linked. Leaders must not only hold others accountable but also accept accountability themselves.

When a process fails or an error occurs, effective leaders avoid blame and instead focus on solutions and learning.

5. Resilience and Adaptability

Healthcare is unpredictable. From pandemics to budget cuts, respiratory leaders must navigate constant change. Resilience is the capacity to bounce back from setbacks; adaptability is the ability to pivot in response to shifting circumstances.

A resilient leader models composure and confidence during crises, which helps maintain team morale. An adaptable leader embraces innovation—whether it's adopting new technologies or reconfiguring workflows in response to staffing shortages.

6. Team Orientation

Leadership is not a solo act. Respiratory leaders succeed when their teams succeed. They invest in building cohesive, collaborative environments where team members feel valued and included.

Team-oriented leaders delegate wisely, foster peer mentorship, and celebrate collective achievements. They recognize that every therapist has unique strengths and seek to leverage them for the greater good.

7. Commitment to Growth

The best leaders are lifelong learners. They seek feedback, pursue continuing education, and reflect critically on their own performance. They also create growth opportunities for others—encouraging therapists to take on new challenges, earn advanced credentials, or participate in quality improvement initiatives.

A commitment to growth also means being humble enough to admit when you don't know something—and curious enough to find out.

BECOMING THE LEADER YOUR TEAM DESERVES

You don't become a great leader by accident. It requires intentional growth, emotional maturity, and the courage to lead through uncertainty. As a respiratory leader, you have the privilege and the responsibility to shape not just clinical outcomes but also human experiences.

The transition from clinician to leader will stretch you. It will challenge your assumptions and push you out of your comfort zone. But in doing so, it offers one of the most meaningful journeys in healthcare: the opportunity to cultivate a culture of excellence that uplifts patients and professionals alike.

DISCUSSION QUESTIONS

- Reflect on a time when you witnessed strong leadership in your department. What specific actions or qualities stood out, and how did they impact the team?
- Which of the key leadership traits do you feel most confident in, and which would you like to develop further? What steps can you take in the next month to strengthen that area?

MODULE TWO

UNDERSTANDING THE HEALTHCARE LANDSCAPE

In today's healthcare environment, effective respiratory leadership requires more than clinical expertise. Leaders must possess a solid understanding of the broader systems in which care is delivered organizational structures, regulatory frameworks, and interprofessional dynamics. This knowledge empowers leaders to align their department's goals with institutional priorities, comply with evolving standards, and foster collaborative care that enhances patient outcomes.

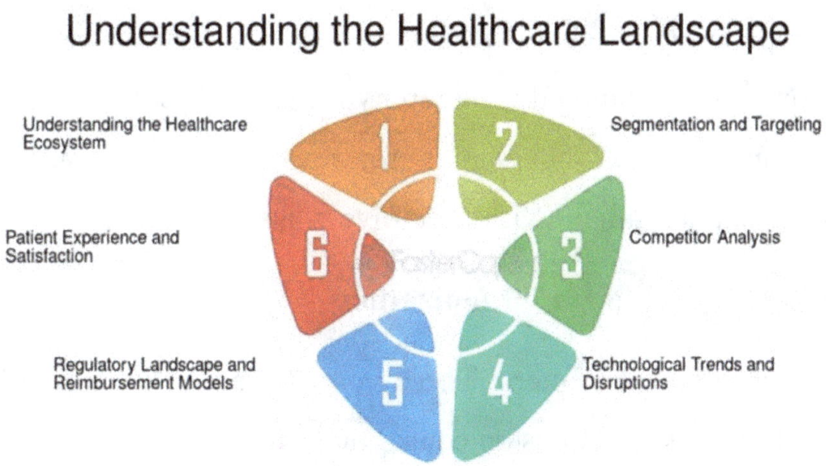

ORGANIZATIONAL STRUCTURES

1. Healthcare System Hierarchies

Healthcare organizations vary in structure, size, and scope, but most follow a hierarchical model with clearly defined roles and reporting lines. At the highest level are executive leaders CEOs, COOs, and CFOs who oversee strategic planning, financial management, and organizational direction. Reporting to them are department heads or service line directors, including those who lead clinical departments such as respiratory therapy, nursing, and radiology.

A respiratory therapy leader typically falls within the clinical operations tier, reporting to a Chief Nursing Officer (CNO), Chief Operating Officer (COO), or directly to a clinical services director. Understanding this hierarchy is essential for navigating institutional politics, advocating for resources, and ensuring departmental alignment with executive goals.

2. Types of Healthcare Organizations

Academic Medical Centers: These hospitals are affiliated with medical schools and focus on education, research, and advanced care. Respiratory leaders in these settings must balance clinical duties with teaching and possibly research initiatives.

- Community Hospitals: These facilities serve local populations and may have smaller respiratory departments. Leaders here often wear multiple hats, managing both clinical and administrative responsibilities.
- Integrated Health Systems: These networks combine multiple care services—acute, ambulatory, post-acute—under one organizational umbrella. Leaders in these systems must understand how respiratory care integrates across various service lines.
- Outpatient and Long-Term Care Facilities: In these environments, respiratory leaders may focus more on chronic care management, home oxygen services, and patient education.

3. Chain of Command and Communication Flow

Understanding the chain of command ensures effective communication, conflict resolution, and escalation of concerns. A respiratory leader must know:

- Who they report to.
- Who reports to them.
- Which committees or task forces require their participation.

- How decisions flow from leadership to staff and vice versa.

This knowledge supports clear communication, avoids duplication of effort, and promotes timely action.

REGULATORY BODIES AND STANDARDS

Healthcare is a heavily regulated field, and respiratory care is governed by multiple agencies and professional organizations that establish standards, ensure quality, and protect patient safety.

1. American Association for Respiratory Care (AARC)

The AARC is the premier professional organization representing respiratory therapists in the U.S. It:

- Sets the scope of practice for RTs.
- Provides clinical practice guidelines (CPGs).
- Offers continuing education and professional development.
- Advocates for the profession at the legislative level.

Leaders should actively engage with the AARC by:

- Encouraging staff membership.
- Promoting credentialing and specialty certifications.

- Aligning department protocols with AARC best practices.

2. The Joint Commission (TJC)

TJC is a nonprofit accreditation body that evaluates healthcare organizations for quality and safety. TJC accreditation is voluntary but essential for credibility and Medicare reimbursement.

For respiratory leaders, TJC standards impact:

- Documentation of assessments and interventions.
- Competency validation and staff training.
- Infection prevention (e.g., equipment sterilization, PPE use).
- Timely administration of respiratory therapies.
- Performance improvement initiatives.

TJC also emphasizes evidence-based care, interdisciplinary communication, and patient-centered practices—all of which align with the mission of respiratory therapy.

1. **3. Centers for Medicare & Medicaid Services (CMS)**

CMS sets national reimbursement standards and regulations for facilities that serve Medicare and Medicaid populations. It plays a key role in determining how respiratory services are coded, billed, and reimbursed.

CMS implications for respiratory leadership include:

- Ensuring respiratory procedures align with CMS-approved services.
- Staying current on respiratory-related quality measures and outcome reporting.
- Leading initiatives that improve value-based care and reduce readmissions.
- Documenting services accurately for proper reimbursement.

4. National Board for Respiratory Care (NBRC)

While not a regulatory agency per se, the NBRC provides credentialing for RTs (e.g., CRT, RRT, and specialty exams such as ACCS, NPS, SDS). Respiratory leaders should:

- Encourage staff to maintain certification.
- Incorporate NBRC competencies into hiring and promotion criteria.
- Use NBRC metrics to guide recruitment and departmental benchmarking.

RESPIRATORY THERAPY'S ROLE IN INTERDISCIPLINARY TEAMS

Respiratory therapists don't work in isolation. They are essential contributors to interdisciplinary care teams that include nurses, physicians, pharmacists, dietitians, and other allied health professionals. Leadership in this space involves more than managing a team, it requires collaboration, communication, and clinical advocacy.

1. Collaborative Care Planning

Respiratory therapists bring specialized knowledge of airway management, oxygen therapy, and mechanical ventilation. In interdisciplinary rounds, they:

- Share input on weaning readiness.
- Recommend treatment adjustments.
- Monitor respiratory status and advocate for escalation or de-escalation.

Leaders must ensure RTs are present and active in these discussions and that their expertise is respected.

2. Clinical Advocacy and Protocol Development

RTs often see patterns and opportunities for improvement before others. Respiratory leaders can:

- Lead development of protocols (e.g., spontaneous breathing trials, bronchodilator weaning).
- Collaborate with physicians on order sets and standing respiratory interventions.
- Represent the RT perspective in policy-making or hospital committees.

This ensures that respiratory therapy is not just reactive but proactive in shaping care delivery.

3. Reducing Silos and Fostering Team Culture

Healthcare has historically suffered from siloed practice nurses, doctors, therapists all operating in separate bubbles. As a leader, you play a vital role in breaking down those silos.

You can:

- Encourage RTs to attend interdisciplinary meetings.
- Facilitate cross-disciplinary in-services or simulations.
- Mediate misunderstandings between disciplines.
- Build mutual respect across professions by highlighting shared goals.

When interdisciplinary teams communicate effectively, patient outcomes improve—and workplace morale rises

4. Supporting Transitions of Care

From ICU to home care, respiratory therapists support patients across the continuum. Leaders must ensure RTs:

- Provide education on inhalers, oxygen use, and respiratory devices at discharge.
- Coordinate with case management and home health providers.
- Document thoroughly to ensure continuity of care and accurate billing.

Leaders can champion initiatives that improve discharge planning and reduce preventable readmissions particularly for patients with COPD, asthma, or post-COVID respiratory complications.

BUILDING SYSTEMS AWARENESS IN LEADERSHIP

Successful respiratory leaders operate with an elevated sense of "systems awareness." This means they understand how decisions made at different organizational levels impact their department and patients. Systems-aware leaders:

- Align departmental goals with hospital strategic plans.
- Advocate for respiratory involvement in organizational initiatives (e.g., sepsis bundles, stroke protocols).

- Monitor performance metrics (e.g., ventilator days, RT response time) and use data to drive improvement.

This broader understanding helps respiratory therapy gain visibility and influence in the larger healthcare arena.

DISCUSSION QUESTIONS

- Which regulatory body or standard has had the most direct impact on how your respiratory department operates? How do you currently engage with or respond to that body's requirements?
- Reflect on an interdisciplinary collaboration you've experienced. What went well, and what could have been improved? How might you, as a leader, strengthen these relationships moving forward?

MODULE THREE

VISION, VALUES, AND CULTURE

A leader's vision and the culture they cultivate are the cornerstones of sustainable excellence in respiratory care. While protocols and procedures provide structure, it is vision and values that give purpose, unify teams, and set the tone for care delivery. This module will explore how respiratory therapy leaders can define a compelling leadership vision, establish core departmental values, and align their efforts with broader hospital-wide goals to build an empowered and high-performing team.

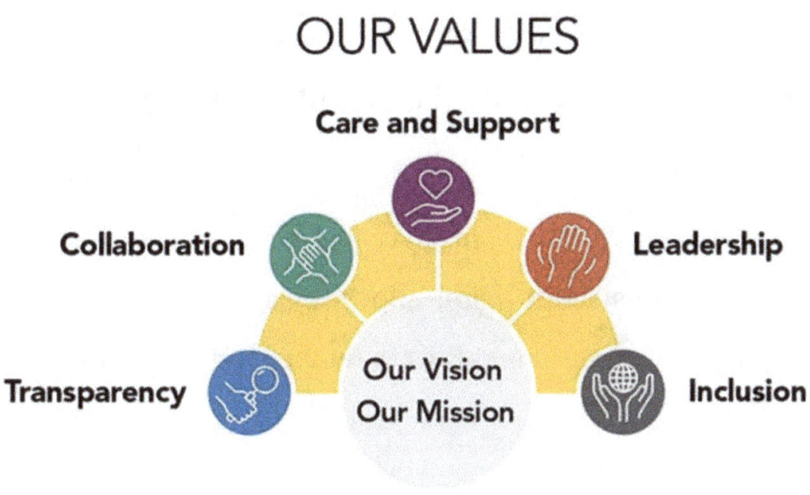

DEFINING YOUR LEADERSHIP VISION

A vision is more than a lofty idea, it is a strategic, forward-looking statement that articulates where your department is headed and why. A well-crafted vision inspires action, fuels engagement, and provides a consistent compass during uncertainty or change.

1. The Purpose of a Leadership Vision

Your vision should:

- Unify your team around a shared future.
- Provide direction when decision-making becomes complex.
- Motivate performance by connecting everyday tasks to meaningful outcomes.
- Communicate leadership identity, showing who you are and what you believe in.

Without a clear vision, teams may feel directionless. In contrast, a clear and consistent vision allows every team member from new graduates to seasoned RTs to understand the "why" behind their work.

2. Crafting Your Vision Statement

When creating a vision, consider the following elements:

- Future-oriented: What will respiratory care look like in your department 3–5 years from now?
- Patient-centered: How will this improve outcomes or the patient experience?
- Team-inclusive: How will your team grow and evolve?
- Aligned: Does it reflect your hospital's mission and strategic plan?

Example Vision Statement:

"To lead respiratory care by fostering innovation, empowering staff, and delivering exceptional, evidence-based respiratory therapy that transforms lives across every patient encounter."

3. Communicating and Living Your Vision

A vision is only useful if it's shared, understood, and reflected in daily practice.

Ways to embed your vision into culture:

- Open every staff meeting with a vision reminder.
- Post the vision in visible staff areas.
- Incorporate it into onboarding, performance reviews, and recognitions.
- Model it consistently in your behavior and decisions.
- Consistency between words and actions builds trust and reinforces the importance of the vision to your team.

ESTABLISHING CORE DEPARTMENTAL VALUES

If the vision answers "Where are we going?", values answer "Who are we as a team?" and "What do we stand for?".

Core values shape the behaviors, attitudes, and priorities of your department. They are the internal compass that guides:

- Clinical decisions
- Team interactions
- Ethical dilemmas
- Hiring and performance standards

1. The Role of Values in Leadership

Values:

- Build team identity and cohesion
- Set expectations for conduct
- Promote psychological safety
- Help leaders navigate conflict and accountability

Without defined values, culture can become reactive or inconsistent. Values ensure your team has a shared moral framework that supports patient care and mutual respect.

2. How to Define Departmental Values

Don't create values in isolation. The most effective values emerge through collaborative dialogue with your team.

Steps to establish values:

- Host a values workshop with staff to brainstorm what matters most in their day-to-day work.
- Identify themes, such as respect, compassion, excellence, integrity, teamwork.
- Define each value clearly, ensuring there's a behavioral component attached.

For example:

Value	**Definition**	**Behavior**
Compassion	We care for patients and each other with empathy and kindness.	We take the time to listen and offer support, especially during stressful moments.
Excellence	We hold ourselves to the highest professional standards.	We stay up to date with current research and pursue continuing education.

3. Embedding Values Into Operations

To make values meaningful, integrate them into:

- Hiring: Select candidates whose behavior aligns with your values.
- Performance reviews: Include value-based behaviors in evaluations.
- Conflict resolution: Use values as a framework for difficult conversations.
- Recognition programs: Reward team members who embody your values.

Example: If "teamwork" is a core value, recognize an RT who supported a nurse during an emergency code, even though they had no obligation to assist.

ALIGNING VALUES WITH HOSPITAL-WIDE GOALS

While departments may have unique roles, all hospital departments must align with larger institutional goals—whether they relate to quality improvement, safety, equity, or financial stewardship. Respiratory leaders serve as a vital bridge between bedside care and organizational strategy.

1. Understanding Institutional Goals

Most hospitals have a strategic plan that includes:

- Mission: Why the hospital exists.
- Vision: What the hospital aspires to become.
- Values: Foundational beliefs and behaviors.
- Key Initiatives: Specific goals for clinical outcomes, safety, patient experience, financial health, etc.

Your department's efforts should echo these priorities. For example, if the hospital aims to reduce readmission rates for COPD patients, your department can:

- Improve discharge education.
- Partner with case managers for follow-up.
- Launch outpatient pulmonary rehab initiatives.

2. Creating a Department Strategy Map

To align your values with broader goals, consider building a departmental strategy map. This document outlines how your team contributes to high-level outcomes.

Example Structure:

Hospital Goal	Department Value	Department Action
Improve patient experience scores	Respect	Train RTs in empathy-based communication.
Reduce hospital-acquired infections	Accountability	Implement new sterilization protocols for respiratory equipment.
Decrease readmission rates	Collaboration	Coordinate care transitions with home health agencies.

Such alignment ensures your team isn't operating in a silo, but rather as a key player in hospital-wide success.

3. Serving as a Culture Carrier

As a leader, you are more than a manager—you are a culture carrier.

You model the vision and values not just in policies, but in how you:

- Speak to staff and patients

- Handle stress or error
- Recognize and reward behavior
- Show up in meetings and committees

Your consistency is key. A leader who talks about excellence but tolerates mediocrity sends a confusing message. Conversely, a leader who models patience, integrity, and motivation sets a standard the team will rise to meet.

Practical Implementation Tips

- Visual Boards: Create vision and values boards in staff break rooms.
- "Values in Action" Spotlights: Feature stories of staff who exemplify your values.
- Monthly Reflection Meetings: Hold brief huddles to discuss how recent decisions or challenges reflect your vision and values.
- Onboarding Culture Moments: Teach new hires about the department's culture on day one.
- Feedback Loops: Encourage staff to reflect on whether the department is living its stated values—and how leadership can do better.

Case Study: Aligning Culture in Action

St. Anne's Medical Center Respiratory Department launched a "Caring in Every Breath" campaign after the department experienced staff burnout and rising patient complaints.

Through several facilitated retreats, the leadership team and frontline RTs co-created a new vision and values statement centered on empathy, responsibility, and innovation. Monthly recognitions, peer-nominated "Culture Champions," and visible leadership presence on the floor helped cement this shift.

Within 12 months:

- Patient satisfaction with respiratory care improved by 28%.
- Voluntary turnover dropped by 35%.
- The department received recognition at a system-wide leadership conference.

Their success illustrates how aligning culture with values and vision is not just abstract—it leads to measurable change.

Vision, values, and culture are not simply buzzwords or soft skills they are strategic assets that shape every outcome in a respiratory department. Leaders who invest time in clarifying and living their vision, involving their team in value creation, and aligning efforts with the broader healthcare system position themselves to lead teams that are resilient, motivated, and deeply impactful.

When respiratory therapy is anchored in vision and guided by shared values, every breath delivered becomes more than just a task it becomes a reflection of purpose.

DISCUSSION QUESTIONS

- What are the current unspoken values in your department, and how do they impact culture, positively or negatively? How would you begin to shift those toward a more intentional set of values?
- Think about a time when a leader's actions contradicted their stated values. How did that affect trust within the team? What lessons can you apply to your own leadership practice?

MODULE FOUR

PSYCHOLOGICAL SAFETY AND TEAM TRUST

A thriving respiratory therapy department doesn't just require clinical expertise—it requires a foundation of trust, open communication, and a culture where individuals feel safe to contribute their ideas, admit mistakes, and grow from challenges. Building a team that works cohesively, communicates openly, and manages conflict productively requires intentional effort. This module will explore how to foster psychological safety in your respiratory department and create an environment of trust where all team members can flourish.

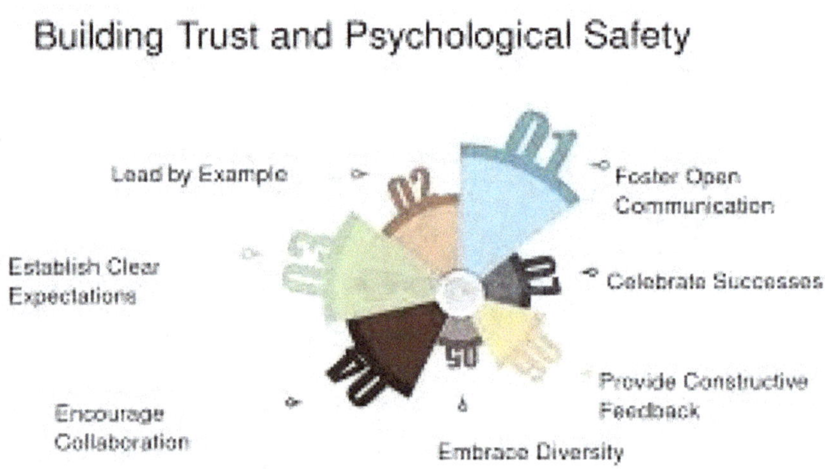
Building Trust and Psychological Safety
Lead by Example
Foster Open Communication
Establish Clear Expectations
Celebrate Successes
Provide Constructive Feedback
Encourage Collaboration
Embrace Diversity
01
02
03
04
05

BUILDING TRUST AMONG TEAM MEMBERS

Trust is the cornerstone of any effective team. Without trust, team members will withhold valuable input, avoid collaboration, and struggle to resolve conflicts productively. In a high-stakes environment like respiratory care, where patient outcomes depend on seamless teamwork, building and maintaining trust is non-negotiable.

1. The Importance of Trust in Respiratory Therapy

In respiratory therapy, trust manifests in various ways:

- Clinical Trust: Team members need to trust each other's clinical competence, knowing that every RT has the skills and knowledge to provide high-quality care.
- Interpersonal Trust: Trusting that colleagues will support each other in stressful moments, collaborate without hesitation, and contribute to team success.
- Emotional Trust: Feeling psychologically safe enough to express vulnerabilities, ask questions, or admit uncertainty without fear of ridicule or backlash.

2. Strategies for Building Trust

1. Model Trust as a Leader As a leader, you must model trust-building behaviors. Trust is often established by the example you set. When you consistently demonstrate honesty,

integrity, and transparency, your team will learn to do the same.

2. Encourage Vulnerability: In a healthcare setting, leaders must create space for their team to be vulnerable. This doesn't mean sharing every personal detail, but it does mean allowing team members to admit when they are unsure, overwhelmed, or need help. When leaders admit mistakes and openly seek feedback, they set a standard for the team.
3. Show Consistency and Reliability: Trust is built through consistent actions. Make sure your actions align with your words, and hold yourself accountable to your commitments. If you say you will follow up on a task, make sure you do it. Being reliable is key to building trust over time.
4. Foster Respect and Inclusion: Encourage all team members to voice their opinions, and ensure that everyone is treated with respect. A diverse and inclusive environment allows for a richer range of perspectives, which can ultimately improve patient care and team effectiveness.
5. Encourage Positive Reinforcement: Recognize and celebrate instances of teamwork and trust-building. Publicly acknowledging when team members demonstrate trustworthiness or collaborate effectively strengthens those behaviors and encourages others to follow suit.

ENCOURAGING OPEN COMMUNICATION

Open communication is the lifeblood of a successful team. In respiratory care, where fast, accurate decision-making is essential, open lines of communication ensure that information flows freely and that there is a shared understanding of the care plan. However, many healthcare teams struggle with communication breakdowns due to hierarchy, time constraints, or fear of conflict.

1. Creating Channels for Open Dialogue

In order to foster open communication, it's important to have both formal and informal channels in place:

- Team Meetings: Regularly scheduled team meetings allow everyone to have a voice and contribute to discussions.
- Informal Check-Ins: Encouraging informal interactions—whether through team huddles, quick conversations in the break room, or virtual platforms—helps maintain continuous communication flow.
- Feedback Mechanisms: Provide anonymous feedback opportunities, like surveys or suggestion boxes, where team members can voice concerns without fear of judgment.

2. Overcoming Communication Barriers

To encourage open communication, it is important to address common barriers, such as:

- Hierarchical Barriers: In many healthcare environments, the chain of command can stifle open communication, particularly when frontline staff feel hesitant to speak to higher-ups. One way to break this down is by implementing an "open-door policy" and encouraging a culture where leadership is accessible.
- Time Constraints: In fast-paced departments like respiratory therapy, time is often a limiting factor. Leaders should set aside specific time for important conversations, even if it means blocking off 10 minutes during shift changes or weekly check-ins.
- Fear of Repercussions: Employees may hesitate to speak openly if they fear their opinions will lead to negative consequences. Leaders can mitigate this by fostering an environment where all feedback is considered valuable, and by handling all input positive and negative with respect.

3. Creating Psychological Safety for Open Dialogue

Psychological safety allows team members to feel safe to speak up, share ideas, and address concerns without the fear of being judged or ridiculed. Leaders can build psychological safety in a number of ways:

- Be Approachable: Establish yourself as a leader who listens actively and responds empathetically.
- Encourage Active Listening: Ensure that when team members speak, they are heard. Encourage reflective listening practices to ensure that all team members' thoughts are understood.
- Reinforce a Culture of Respect: Promote an atmosphere where differences in opinion are welcomed and addressed constructively, rather than shutting down dissenting views.
- Normalize Mistakes: Remind your team that mistakes are part of learning and growing. By doing so, you reduce the fear of failure and encourage team members to speak up about potential issues before they become bigger problems.

MANAGING CONFLICT PRODUCTIVELY

Conflict is inevitable in any team setting. In healthcare, it can arise due to differences in clinical judgment, personality clashes, workload stress, or miscommunication. While unresolved conflict can disrupt teamwork and compromise patient care, when managed properly, conflict can become a powerful tool for improvement and growth.

1. Recognizing Healthy vs. Unhealthy Conflict

Healthy Conflict:

- Occurs when team members express differing views constructively.
- Focuses on solving problems or improving processes.
- Is dealt with promptly, keeping the focus on the issue, not personal attacks.

Unhealthy Conflict:

- Involves hostility, personal attacks, or resentment.
- Is prolonged and unresolved, leading to division within the team.
- Disrupts communication and may negatively impact patient care.

2. Techniques for Managing Conflict

- Encourage Early Intervention: Leaders should encourage their teams to address conflicts as soon as they arise, rather than letting issues fester. Early intervention can prevent small misunderstandings from escalating into major problems.

- Listen to All Sides: When conflict arises, make sure to listen to all parties involved. Avoid taking sides or making assumptions. Rather than focusing solely on finding a quick resolution, try to understand the perspectives of each person involved.
- Focus on the Issue, Not the Person: When addressing conflict, always keep the focus on the issue at hand, not the individuals involved. This encourages constructive dialogue and minimizes personal attacks. Instead of asking "Why did you do that?", ask "How can we solve this together?"
- Find Common Ground: In any conflict, identifying shared goals is crucial. In respiratory care, the common goal is always patient well-being. By focusing on the mutual objective of delivering the best possible care, team members are more likely to find common ground and work collaboratively.
- Encourage Collaboration, Not Competition: Create an environment where collaboration is valued over competition. Encourage team members to work together to solve problems rather than focusing on being "right."
- Role of the Leader in Conflict Resolution: As a leader, your role is to mediate conflict and guide the team toward resolution. Avoid being the sole decision-maker; instead, empower team members to discuss and decide on the

solution collaboratively. By doing so, you promote shared ownership of both the conflict and its resolution.

Building trust, encouraging open communication, and managing conflict productively are all critical components of a high-functioning respiratory therapy team. These elements work together to create a psychologically safe environment where team members feel valued, heard, and supported. In a healthcare setting, where patient outcomes depend on collaboration and quick, efficient decision-making, fostering these qualities is essential to both clinical success and employee satisfaction.

By intentionally building trust, fostering open dialogue, and addressing conflict in a constructive manner, respiratory therapy leaders can create a culture where team members thrive, patients benefit, and excellence becomes the standard.

DISCUSSION QUESTIONS

- Reflect on a time when open communication or trust was lacking within a healthcare team. What were the consequences, and what steps could have been taken to improve the situation?
- How do you, as a leader, currently handle conflict in your team? What changes could you implement to ensure that conflict is addressed productively and doesn't affect team morale?

MODULE FIVE

MOTIVATION THAT LASTS

In the fast-paced world of respiratory therapy, where every decision impacts patient care, keeping your team motivated is a fundamental part of effective leadership. As a respiratory leader, your role goes beyond managing workflows and ensuring compliance with regulations you must inspire, encourage, and sustain motivation within your team to foster an environment of excellence.

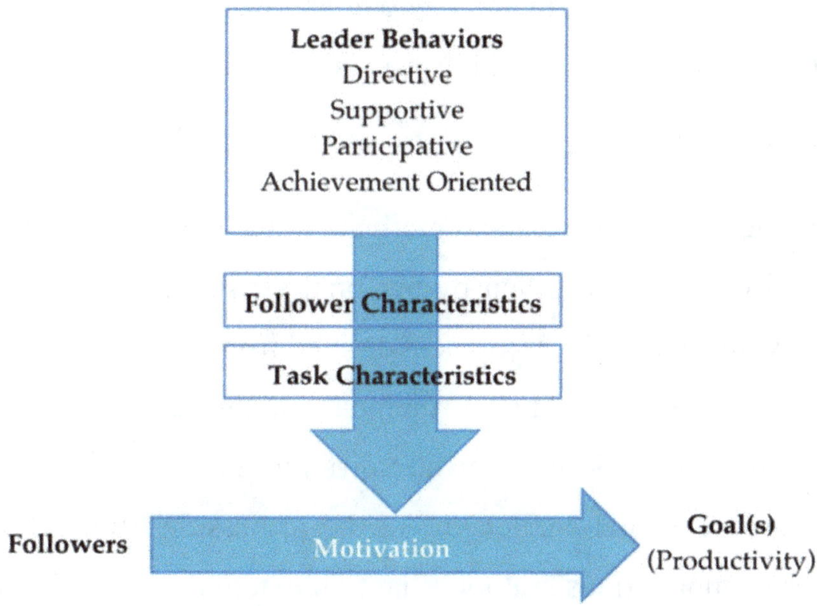

Motivation is often the key difference between high-performing teams and those that simply get by. But how can you create motivation that lasts, especially in a field that is physically and emotionally demanding? This module will explore the dynamics of intrinsic versus extrinsic motivation, recognition and reward strategies, and leading through inspiration instead of intimidation to cultivate long-term engagement and satisfaction within your respiratory therapy department.

INTRINSIC VS. EXTRINSIC MOTIVATION

Motivation, at its core, is what drives individuals to act, persist, and perform at their best. It's what gets your team to go the extra mile, handle high-pressure situations, and continue delivering exceptional care day in and day out. Motivation can be divided into two broad categories: intrinsic and extrinsic.

1. Intrinsic Motivation

Intrinsic motivation refers to motivation that comes from within an individual. It is driven by personal satisfaction, a sense of achievement, and the enjoyment derived from the activity itself. For example, a respiratory therapist might feel intrinsically motivated by the desire to make a difference in patients' lives or by the intellectual challenge that the profession offers. These types of motivations are not reliant on external rewards but are fueled by internal desires.

Key Characteristics of Intrinsic Motivation:

- Autonomy: The desire to work independently and have control over one's tasks.
- Mastery: The pursuit of improvement and the satisfaction of developing one's skills and expertise.
- Purpose: A sense of contributing to a greater cause or mission, such as improving patient outcomes or being part of a team that strives for excellence.

How to Foster Intrinsic Motivation:

- Empower Your Team: Allow team members to take ownership of their work and have the autonomy to make decisions about patient care or team initiatives.
- Create Opportunities for Growth: Encourage continuous learning and skill development through education, mentorship, and training. Help team members set personal goals and pursue professional certifications.
- Connect Work to a Larger Purpose: Remind team members of the importance of their work in the context of patient care and how their efforts contribute to the hospital's mission and the broader healthcare system.

2. Extrinsic Motivation

Extrinsic motivation, on the other hand, comes from external factors. It is driven by tangible rewards such as pay, bonuses, promotions, or public recognition. While extrinsic motivation can be effective in driving short-term results or motivating individuals to meet specific goals, it is not sustainable in the long term unless it is linked to intrinsic motivators.

Key Characteristics of Extrinsic Motivation:

- External Rewards: Tangible incentives such as money, promotions, or recognition.
- Performance-Oriented: Motivated by meeting measurable outcomes or meeting deadlines.
- Task-Oriented: Focused on completing specific tasks for external validation or approval.

Balancing Intrinsic and Extrinsic Motivation:

- Avoid Over-Reliance on External Rewards: While recognition and rewards are important, over-relying on them can lead to burnout or a lack of long-term engagement. Ensure that intrinsic factors like personal growth, purpose, and mastery are cultivated alongside extrinsic rewards.
- Tailor Rewards to Individuals: Not all team members are motivated by the same extrinsic rewards. While one individual may be motivated by public recognition, another may prefer a more private acknowledgment or a financial incentive. It's important to understand what motivates each team member on an individual level.

RECOGNITION AND REWARD STRATEGIES

Recognition and reward are powerful tools for sustaining motivation. By acknowledging team members' efforts, you not only validate their hard work but also reinforce the behaviors and outcomes you wish to see more of in the future.

1. The Importance of Recognition

Recognition makes team members feel valued, appreciated, and seen for their contributions. It boosts morale and creates a positive work environment. According to research, employees who feel appreciated are more likely to be engaged, stay with the organization, and perform at higher levels.

Types of Recognition:

- Public Recognition: Acknowledging team members in front of peers, whether in team meetings or through hospital-wide communications. This type of recognition can build pride and encourage friendly competition.
- Private Recognition: Offering one-on-one praise or a personal note of appreciation. Some individuals may prefer private recognition to avoid attention, but it is just as meaningful and powerful.

- Peer Recognition: Encouraging team members to recognize one another's contributions can foster a sense of camaraderie and unity within the team.

2. Rewarding Your Team

While recognition is about showing appreciation, rewards are tangible incentives that can enhance motivation, particularly for extrinsically motivated individuals. However, rewards should be tied to meaningful achievements and not just routine tasks to avoid devaluing their significance.

Types of Rewards:

- Financial Rewards: Pay raises, bonuses, and incentive programs are often the most direct form of reward. However, these should be used thoughtfully, as over-relying on financial incentives can undermine intrinsic motivation.
- Non-Financial Rewards: Consider offering rewards that promote work-life balance, such as extra time off, flexible scheduling, or access to wellness programs.
- Career Development Rewards: Providing opportunities for career advancement, education, and training is a powerful way to reward employees and further nurture their intrinsic motivation.

3. Creating a Recognition-Rich Culture

For recognition and reward strategies to be effective, they must be a regular part of the team culture, not just something that occurs on rare occasions. Consistent acknowledgment of both individual and team achievements helps to foster a sense of accomplishment and purpose among all staff members.

- Create a Recognition Program: Develop a formal recognition program where employees are nominated by peers or managers for going above and beyond in their work. Recognize not just exceptional performance, but also efforts to improve team dynamics, patient care, and departmental innovation.
- Regular Feedback: Foster a culture of continuous feedback, where praise and constructive criticism are given regularly. This helps maintain engagement and ensures team members know how they are doing and where they can improve.
- Celebrate Team Achievements: Recognize the collective achievements of the team, whether it's reaching a departmental goal, improving patient outcomes, or completing a successful project. Celebrating team success strengthens bonds and builds morale.

LEADING THROUGH INSPIRATION, NOT INTIMIDATION

Effective leadership in respiratory therapy requires the ability to inspire and motivate rather than relying on fear-based tactics. Leaders who use intimidation may achieve short-term compliance, but they risk stifling creativity, reducing team cohesion, and fostering resentment. In contrast, leaders who inspire foster an environment where team members are motivated by shared vision, personal growth, and a sense of purpose.

1. Inspiring, Not Intimidating

Leaders who lead by inspiration create an atmosphere of trust, collaboration, and shared responsibility. These leaders:

- Lead by Example: They model the behaviors they expect from their team, whether it's punctuality, professionalism, or a commitment to patient care.
- Empower Others: They encourage their team members to take ownership of their work, make decisions, and contribute to the department's success.
- Encourage Creativity and Innovation: Leaders who inspire welcome new ideas, innovations, and improvements. They see mistakes as learning

opportunities rather than failures, which motivates their team to be bold and think outside the box.

2. Avoiding Intimidation Tactics

Intimidation tactics often involve fear-based leadership where the leader instills fear of consequences, retribution, or failure. While these tactics may result in short-term compliance, they can lead to higher employee turnover, burnout, and a lack of creativity.

Instead of intimidation, it's crucial to build relationships of trust and mutual respect. Acknowledge your team members' contributions, provide constructive feedback, and address concerns with empathy.

3. Building an Inspiring Vision

An inspiring leader has a clear vision for the department and communicates this vision to the team. By aligning the team's individual goals with the broader goals of the department or hospital, you can create a sense of purpose that drives sustained motivation.

Key Strategies for Building and Communicating a Vision:

- Communicate the "Why": Leaders who inspire clearly articulate the purpose behind the work being done. For example, in respiratory therapy, you can emphasize the impact your department has on patient recovery and well-being.

- Set Challenging but Achievable Goals: Provide opportunities for team members to grow and push their limits, but ensure the goals are realistic and achievable.
- Foster a Positive Team Culture: Inspire a positive team culture that emphasizes collaboration, support, and mutual respect. A positive work environment leads to intrinsic motivation and long-term satisfaction.

Motivation is a critical component of effective leadership in respiratory therapy. By understanding the dynamics between intrinsic and extrinsic motivation, implementing effective recognition and reward strategies, and leading through inspiration instead of intimidation, you can build a motivated, engaged, and high-performing team. The motivation you cultivate within your team will have a direct impact on patient care, job satisfaction, and overall departmental success.

DISCUSSION QUESTIONS

- What intrinsic motivators do you believe are most important in your department, and how can you cultivate these within your team?

- Reflecting on your leadership style, do you tend to lead more by inspiration or intimidation? How can you adjust your approach to inspire your team more effectively?

MODULE SIX

ACCOUNTABILITY IN ACTION

Accountability is an essential element in any team-oriented environment, and in healthcare, it becomes even more crucial. For respiratory therapy departments, where patient outcomes depend on a collaborative approach and precise execution of complex tasks, accountability ensures that everyone understands their roles, works to meet objectives, and consistently delivers quality care. This module will explore how to set expectations and measurable goals, implement effective feedback loops, and coach underperformers with compassion and clarity. These strategies will foster a culture of accountability that drives both personal and team-wide success.

Ensuring Accountability at the Leadership Level

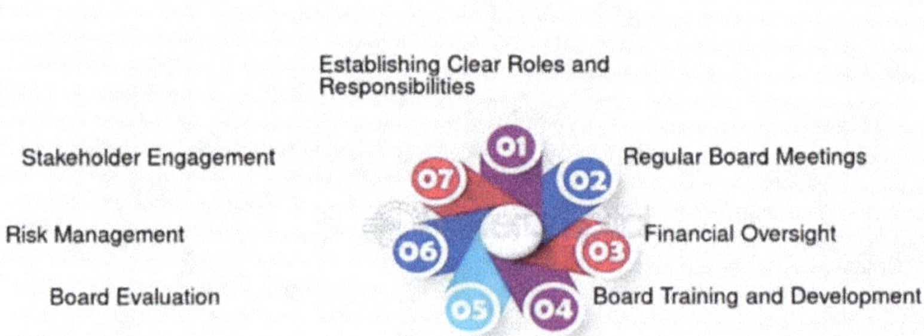

SETTING EXPECTATIONS AND MEASURABLE GOALS

Clear expectations and measurable goals are fundamental to fostering a culture of accountability in any department. Without a clear understanding of what is expected, employees may feel confused, overwhelmed, or unmotivated. On the other hand, well-defined goals provide direction and help team members focus their efforts toward common objectives, all while reinforcing accountability.

1. Setting Clear Expectations

Expectations should be set early and communicated clearly to all team members. A well-established framework of expectations helps eliminate ambiguity and ensures everyone is on the same page.

Key Components of Setting Expectations:

- Job Roles and Responsibilities: Each team member must understand their specific duties and how they contribute to the overall functioning of the department. This includes both clinical duties (e.g., administering respiratory therapy treatments) and non-clinical duties (e.g., documentation, patient education).

- Behavioral Expectations: Along with performance expectations, it's important to establish behavioral norms that promote collaboration, professionalism, and respect within the team.
- Standards of Care: Establish clear expectations surrounding the quality of care your department is committed to providing. This includes adhering to established protocols, safety measures, and patient care standards.
- Departmental Goals: These should align with the hospital's overall goals, emphasizing patient satisfaction, treatment outcomes, compliance with regulations, and efficiency in workflow.

How to Communicate Expectations Effectively:

- Clear and Concise: Ensure that expectations are communicated in a way that is simple, clear, and free from jargon. This may involve written documents, verbal explanations, and demonstrations.
- Frequent Check-ins: Regular meetings and check-ins allow for clarification of any questions or concerns regarding expectations.
- Ensure Alignment: Verify that all team members understand how their individual goals align with

departmental and organizational goals. When everyone is aware of their role in achieving broader objectives, they are more likely to stay motivated and accountable.

2. Measurable Goals

Setting measurable goals enables you to track progress and determine whether the team is meeting its objectives. These goals should be specific, attainable, and relevant to the department's overarching mission.

Characteristics of Effective Measurable Goals:

- Specific: Goals should be clear and specific, focusing on concrete outcomes (e.g., reducing patient recovery time, increasing the number of completed therapy sessions per week).
- Measurable: There should be clear criteria for success, such as performance metrics (e.g., compliance with protocols, patient satisfaction scores, or improved clinical outcomes).
- Achievable: While goals should be challenging, they must also be realistic and within the team's capacity to achieve, given available resources and time.
- Relevant: Goals should align with the department's needs and priorities, as well as the hospital's overall strategic objectives.

- Time-Bound: Setting a timeline ensures that goals are pursued with a sense of urgency and helps track progress over time.

How to Set Measurable Goals:

- SMART Goals Framework: Use the SMART criteria (Specific, Measurable, Achievable, Relevant, and Time-bound) to ensure that the goals you set are well-structured.
- Data-Driven Metrics: Rely on objective data to set your goals. For example, you can use past performance metrics, patient feedback, or industry standards to identify areas for improvement and target specific outcomes.
- Engage Your Team in Goal Setting: Involve team members in the goal-setting process. This increases their investment in achieving the goals and fosters a sense of ownership.

IMPLEMENTING EFFECTIVE FEEDBACK LOOPS

Effective feedback is a critical component of maintaining accountability and driving continuous improvement. It allows employees to understand how well they are performing, where they can improve, and how they can contribute more effectively to the team's success.

1. The Importance of Feedback

Feedback is a powerful tool that enhances personal and professional growth. When given constructively, it helps individuals identify strengths and weaknesses, correct mistakes, and refine skills. In the context of a respiratory therapy department, feedback helps ensure that quality care is being delivered and that standards are upheld.

The Role of Feedback in Accountability:

- Reinforces Expectations: Feedback helps remind team members of what is expected and reinforces the behaviors and actions that align with departmental goals.
- Improves Performance: Constructive feedback highlights areas for improvement, ensuring that the team continually raises its standards and enhances the quality of patient care.
- Strengthens Team Morale: Regular, balanced feedback (both positive and constructive) builds trust and morale. Employees who feel recognized for their contributions are more likely to stay engaged and motivated.

2. Providing Constructive Feedback

Constructive feedback should focus on specific behaviors or outcomes, rather than generalizations. It should aim to improve performance without diminishing the individual's confidence or self-esteem.

Key Elements of Constructive Feedback:

- Timeliness: Feedback should be given in a timely manner, close to the event or performance being evaluated. This ensures it is relevant and allows for immediate correction if necessary.
- Specificity: Focus on specific actions or behaviors, not on the person as a whole. For example, instead of saying "You did a poor job," say "The documentation for this case was incomplete, and we need to ensure all details are recorded accurately."
- Balance: Provide both positive and constructive feedback. Acknowledge what has been done well before addressing areas for improvement. This approach prevents the team member from feeling discouraged and helps maintain morale.
- Actionable Suggestions: Feedback should include actionable steps for improvement, so the individual knows exactly what they can do to enhance their performance in the future.

3. Creating a Feedback Culture

A culture of continuous feedback is essential for fostering accountability. When feedback is encouraged, not just during annual performance reviews but on a regular basis, it becomes a tool for growth rather than a source of anxiety.

Strategies to Foster a Feedback Culture:

- Regular Check-ins: Schedule routine one-on-one meetings to discuss performance and provide feedback. These sessions should be opportunities for open dialogue, where the team member feels comfortable asking questions and expressing concerns.
- Peer-to-Peer Feedback: Encourage a culture of peer feedback, where colleagues provide constructive insights to each other. This strengthens relationships and ensures that team members hold each other accountable.
- Feedback Training: Train managers and team members on how to give and receive feedback effectively. Teaching employees how to deliver feedback in a respectful and constructive manner ensures that it's productive and beneficial.

COACHING UNDERPERFORMERS WITH COMPASSION AND CLARITY

Not every team member will perform at their best all the time. When dealing with underperformance, it's important to approach the situation with compassion and clarity, ensuring that feedback is received in a positive manner and that the individual is given the tools they need to improve.

1. Understanding the Root Cause of Underperformance

Before coaching an underperformer, it's essential to understand the root cause of the issue. There could be many reasons for underperformance, including personal challenges, unclear expectations, lack of training, or lack of motivation.

Steps to Diagnose Underperformance:

- Assess Performance Data: Review specific metrics, such as patient outcomes, compliance with protocols, or feedback from peers and supervisors. Identifying patterns can help pinpoint where the underperformance is occurring.
- One-on-One Conversations: Have an open, empathetic conversation with the team member to understand any challenges they are facing. Ask open-ended questions to encourage dialogue and make them feel heard.

- Offer Support and Resources: If training or resources are needed, ensure that they are provided. Sometimes underperformance is due to a lack of necessary skills or tools.

2. Coaching with Compassion and Clarity

When addressing underperformance, it's important to balance clarity with empathy. The goal is to provide the individual with actionable steps for improvement while maintaining their dignity and morale.

Key Principles for Coaching Underperformers:

- Be Compassionate: Approach the conversation with empathy, understanding that everyone faces challenges and setbacks. Avoid making the individual feel ashamed or defensive.
- Set Clear Expectations for Improvement: Clearly articulate the areas where performance needs to improve, and outline specific actions the team member can take. Offer support to help them reach their goals.
- Offer Continuous Support: Coaching doesn't end with a single conversation. Offer ongoing feedback, check-ins, and encouragement to ensure progress is being made.
- Follow-up: Schedule follow-up meetings to review progress and provide additional feedback. If performance

improves, acknowledge the effort and reinforce positive changes.

3. Building Confidence Through Coaching

Coaching is not just about pointing out flaws; it's about helping individuals build confidence in their abilities. By providing clear expectations, offering resources for development, and giving regular feedback, leaders can help team members become more self-assured and motivated to perform at their best.

Accountability is the backbone of any high-functioning respiratory therapy department. By setting clear expectations, establishing measurable goals, implementing effective feedback loops, and coaching underperformers with compassion and clarity, leaders can foster a culture of accountability that drives continuous improvement. A department that is held accountable is more likely to achieve its objectives, enhance patient care, and create a positive work environment for its team members.

DISCUSSION QUESTIONS

- How can you ensure that all team members clearly understand expectations and goals within your department? What strategies have you found most effective?

- When coaching underperformers, how can you strike the right balance between empathy and holding them accountable for their performance?

MODULE SEVEN

STAFF DEVELOPMENT AND RETENTION

The healthcare industry, especially in specialized fields like respiratory therapy, faces a constant challenge: maintaining a well-trained, motivated, and committed workforce. Retaining highly skilled professionals is just as crucial as recruiting them. Respiratory therapy departments must not only focus on providing high-quality care but also invest in the professional development of their staff to keep them engaged, motivated, and capable of meeting the demands of a dynamic healthcare environment. This module explores key strategies for staff development and retention, including creating development plans, mentorship and peer coaching, and preventing burnout while promoting well-being.

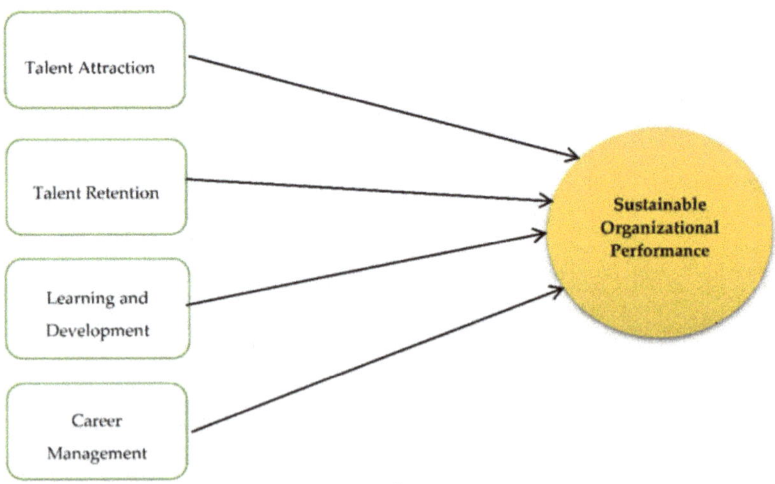

CREATING DEVELOPMENT PLANS

Development plans are essential tools in any healthcare department for fostering staff growth, satisfaction, and retention. These plans provide staff members with clear pathways for advancement and skill development, which can lead to increased job satisfaction, improved performance, and reduced turnover rates.

1. Why Development Plans Matter

In a rapidly evolving healthcare landscape, respiratory therapists need to continuously upgrade their knowledge and skills to keep pace with new treatments, technology, and regulatory requirements. A well-structured development plan helps to guide individual progress and create a roadmap for career advancement.

Benefits of Development Plans:

- Enhance Job Satisfaction: Employees are more likely to stay in positions where they feel they are growing personally and professionally.
- Boost Professional Competency: Through ongoing development, staff members stay abreast of the latest respiratory care practices, which leads to improved patient outcomes.

- Support Organizational Goals: Development plans help align the personal goals of the staff with departmental and organizational objectives, ensuring that the team works toward a common purpose.
- Improve Retention: Employees are more likely to remain in organizations that invest in their future and provide opportunities for growth.

2. How to Create Effective Development Plans

A well-crafted development plan includes specific goals, actionable steps, and a timeline for achieving these objectives. It should be tailored to the individual's needs, career aspirations, and the demands of the department.

Key Elements of a Development Plan:

- Individualized Goals: Assess the individual's strengths, weaknesses, and career goals. Discuss with the team member what they want to achieve in the short-term and long-term.
- Skill Development: Identify key skills that need to be developed. For respiratory therapists, this might include advanced technical competencies, leadership skills, or a deeper understanding of clinical protocols.

- Training and Education: Provide access to ongoing education, such as certification programs, workshops, conferences, or formal academic courses.
- Mentorship: Ensure there is a mentor or senior therapist who can offer guidance, advice, and support as the team member progresses.
- Progress Review: Regularly review the development plan to track progress, make adjustments if needed, and celebrate achievements. This could be in the form of quarterly check-ins or annual performance reviews.

3. Measuring Success

Development plans should have measurable outcomes. These can include tangible skills gained, certifications achieved, leadership roles undertaken, or clinical outcomes improved. Tracking the completion of goals ensures that the staff member is progressing and that their professional growth is aligned with the department's objectives.

MENTORSHIP AND PEER COACHING

Mentorship and peer coaching are powerful tools in staff development and retention. These strategies provide opportunities for less experienced staff members to learn from their more experienced colleagues and build supportive relationships that enhance professional growth.

1. The Role of Mentorship

Mentorship is a structured relationship where a more experienced therapist (the mentor) provides guidance and support to a less experienced team member (the mentee). This relationship can be formal or informal, but its core purpose is to help the mentee grow professionally.

Benefits of Mentorship:

- Career Advancement: Mentors can provide advice on how to navigate career challenges, expand professional networks, and identify new opportunities.
- Increased Confidence: A mentor's support helps mentees build confidence in their clinical and leadership abilities.
- Enhanced Job Satisfaction: Mentees who receive mentorship are more likely to feel valued and supported, which enhances their overall job satisfaction and loyalty.
- Stronger Departmental Culture: Mentorship fosters a culture of collaboration, knowledge-sharing, and teamwork, essential for a high-performing respiratory therapy department.

2. Peer Coaching

Peer coaching is a less formal but equally effective method for developing staff. In this model, colleagues who are at similar levels of experience work together to support each other's development. Peer coaching allows for collaborative learning and can be particularly beneficial in a dynamic healthcare setting where team-based care is paramount.

Benefits of Peer Coaching:

- Improved Communication: Peer coaching fosters open communication and collaboration, which enhances overall team performance.
- Reinforced Learning: By discussing cases, challenges, and techniques with peers, staff members can reinforce their learning and clarify doubts.
- Increased Accountability: Peer coaching encourages mutual accountability, as both individuals are invested in each other's development and success.
- Fostering a Positive Team Culture: It builds a sense of camaraderie and support among colleagues, strengthening relationships within the team.

3. Implementing a Mentorship and Peer Coaching Program

To establish a formal mentorship or peer coaching program, the following steps should be taken:

- Identify Potential Mentors and Coaches: Choose experienced, respected staff members who have the necessary skills and qualities to guide others.
- Define Goals and Expectations: Set clear expectations for both mentors and mentees or coaches, outlining the purpose and structure of the relationship.
- Provide Support and Resources: Offer training on how to mentor or coach effectively and ensure that both mentors and mentees have access to resources for continuous learning.
- Regular Check-ins: Ensure that mentorship and coaching relationships are regularly evaluated to monitor progress and address any challenges.

PREVENTING BURNOUT AND PROMOTING WELL-BEING

Healthcare professionals, especially in high-stress environments like respiratory therapy, are vulnerable to burnout. Burnout is a state of emotional, physical, and mental exhaustion caused by excessive and prolonged stress, and it can significantly impact both the individual's well-being and the quality of patient care. Preventing burnout and promoting well-being should be integral to any staff development and retention strategy.

1. Understanding Burnout

Burnout manifests as emotional exhaustion, depersonalization (feeling detached from work or patients), and a reduced sense of personal accomplishment. Respiratory therapists are at high risk for burnout due to the emotionally intense nature of their work, long shifts, and constant exposure to critical care situations.

Risk Factors for Burnout:

- Workload: High patient caseloads and the demand for constant care can contribute to physical and emotional exhaustion.
- Lack of Control: Feeling powerless or lacking control over decisions can lead to frustration and burnout.
- Lack of Support: Without sufficient mentorship, feedback, and collegial support, staff may feel isolated and overwhelmed.
- Unresolved Conflict: Tension and unresolved conflict within the team can erode morale and contribute to stress.

2. Strategies for Preventing Burnout

To combat burnout, departments must take proactive measures that support the mental and physical well-being of their staff.

Key Strategies for Preventing Burnout:

- Work-Life Balance: Encourage employees to take regular breaks, use their vacation time, and disconnect from work during their off-hours. Promote the importance of setting boundaries between personal and professional life.
- Flexible Scheduling: Offering flexible work schedules can help employees manage personal obligations and reduce stress.
- Employee Assistance Programs (EAP): Implement programs that provide counseling, mental health resources, and wellness support.
- Supportive Leadership: Leaders should actively engage with their teams, provide regular feedback, and ensure that staff feel valued and supported.
- Recognize Achievements: Recognizing and celebrating achievements, whether big or small, can boost morale and reduce stress.
- Promote Physical Health: Encourage physical wellness programs, such as fitness challenges, yoga, or mindfulness sessions, to help staff maintain physical and emotional health.

3. Promoting Well-being

Beyond preventing burnout, it's crucial to create a culture of well-being where staff members feel their overall health and happiness are prioritized.

Well-being Strategies:

- Mental Health Support: Provide access to mental health resources, such as counseling or stress management workshops, and reduce the stigma associated with seeking help.
- Team Building: Foster team-building activities that allow staff to unwind, relax, and build positive relationships outside of the work environment.
- Encourage Self-Care: Educate staff on the importance of self-care and offer resources on how to incorporate it into their daily routines.
- Create a Positive Work Environment: Ensure that the work environment is supportive, collaborative, and free from toxic behaviors that can contribute to stress.

Staff development and retention are critical to the success of any respiratory therapy department. By creating development plans, promoting mentorship and peer coaching, and actively working to prevent burnout while supporting well-being, leaders can ensure their team members are motivated, satisfied, and equipped to provide the highest level of care. When staff feel valued and supported, they are more likely to stay engaged, develop professionally, and remain committed to their roles, leading to improved patient outcomes and a thriving department.

DISCUSSION QUESTIONS

- What strategies have you found most effective in promoting staff development in your department? How do you ensure that the development plans align with both individual goals and departmental needs?
- In what ways can you foster a culture of well-being in your department that reduces burnout and supports staff members' overall health and happiness?

MODULE EIGHT

QUALITY IMPROVEMENT AND EVIDENCE-BASED PRACTICE

In today's healthcare environment, delivering the highest quality of care is non-negotiable. Respiratory therapy departments, like any other part of the healthcare system, must ensure that the care provided is not only effective but also efficient, safe, and continuously improving. The concepts of quality improvement (QI) and evidence-based practice (EBP) play a pivotal role in achieving these goals. This module explores these two key concepts in depth, particularly as they apply to respiratory care. It will also examine the use of Key Performance Indicators (KPIs), Lean and Six Sigma methodologies, and strategies for creating a continuous improvement mindset.

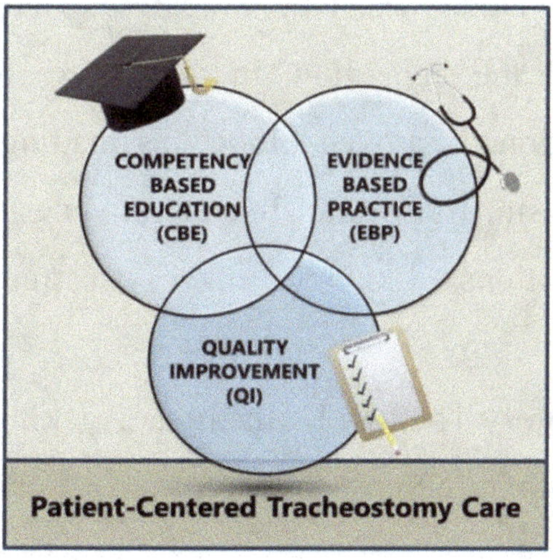

UNDERSTANDING KPIS IN RESPIRATORY CARE

1. What are KPIs?

Key Performance Indicators (KPIs) are quantifiable measures used to evaluate the effectiveness of an organization, department, or individual in achieving a specific objective. In the context of respiratory care, KPIs allow respiratory therapy departments to assess the quality of care provided, monitor patient outcomes, and ensure that care is delivered in a timely and cost-effective manner.

Key KPIs in Respiratory Care:

- Patient Satisfaction: Monitoring patient satisfaction through surveys or feedback forms helps ensure that respiratory services meet patient expectations and contribute to a positive care experience.
- Clinical Outcomes: Key indicators of clinical outcomes include the reduction in the need for mechanical ventilation, improved blood gas readings, reduction in readmission rates, and the effectiveness of therapeutic interventions like nebulizer treatments or chest physiotherapy.
- Respiratory Therapy Utilization: Tracking the number of respiratory therapy interventions, consultations, and

procedures performed during a given period can provide insight into resource utilization.

- Compliance with Clinical Guidelines: Respiratory care departments must ensure that evidence-based guidelines for managing conditions like COPD, asthma, or pneumonia are consistently followed. KPIs can be used to monitor compliance rates.
- Staff Efficiency: KPIs like response time to calls, number of patients seen per shift, and patient throughput can measure staff efficiency and workload management.

2. How KPIs Improve Respiratory Care

KPIs serve several important functions in respiratory care:

- Benchmarking Performance: KPIs provide measurable benchmarks for departments to assess their performance over time or in comparison to industry standards.
- Improving Decision-Making: Data collected from KPIs can guide decisions on resource allocation, staffing, training, and process improvements.
- Identifying Areas for Improvement: KPIs highlight areas where performance is lacking, prompting corrective actions to enhance quality and patient outcomes.
- Encouraging Accountability: KPIs hold staff members and departments accountable for maintaining high

standards of care, improving efficiency, and adhering to protocols.

3. Developing and Implementing KPIs

To develop KPIs that are meaningful and useful for respiratory care departments, leaders must work closely with clinical teams to ensure that the measures are relevant to their specific context. The following steps should be taken:

- Identify Department Goals: What are the main objectives of the department? These goals might include improving patient outcomes, reducing readmission rates, or optimizing resource use.
- Set Specific, Measurable, Achievable, Relevant, and Time-bound (SMART) Targets: Ensure KPIs are aligned with the department's broader goals and that they meet the SMART criteria.
- Monitor and Evaluate: Continuously track and review KPIs to ensure that they provide an accurate picture of departmental performance and patient outcomes.
- Adjust as Needed: KPIs should be reviewed and adjusted regularly to ensure they remain relevant and accurately reflect the evolving goals of the department.

LEAN AND SIX SIGMA IN HEALTHCARE

1. What are Lean and Six Sigma?

Lean and Six Sigma are two process improvement methodologies that focus on increasing efficiency, reducing waste, and improving quality. Both have their roots in manufacturing but have been successfully applied to healthcare settings to enhance the quality of care and improve operational effectiveness.

Lean: Lean focuses on streamlining processes by identifying and eliminating waste, improving flow, and maximizing value for both patients and healthcare providers.

Six Sigma: Six Sigma aims to reduce variability in processes by identifying defects, measuring their impact, and using statistical methods to control and improve processes.

Both methodologies can be used in tandem, with Lean focusing on eliminating waste and Six Sigma focusing on reducing defects and improving consistency.

2. Applying Lean in Respiratory Care

In respiratory therapy, Lean can be used to identify inefficiencies in the care process, from patient intake to discharge. Waste can come in many forms, such as unnecessary steps in care delivery, delays in treatments, or excessive use of resources.

Key Lean Principles in Respiratory Therapy:

- Value Stream Mapping: This tool is used to visualize the entire patient care process, from the moment they enter the hospital to discharge. This helps identify areas where there are delays, redundancies, or inefficiencies.
- Eliminating Waste: Lean focuses on reducing seven types of waste, including excess motion, waiting times, overproduction, inventory, defects, and unnecessary transportation.
- Standardizing Work: By standardizing procedures for common respiratory treatments, such as nebulizer therapy or oxygen administration, departments can reduce variability and improve efficiency.

3. Applying Six Sigma in Respiratory Care

Six Sigma focuses on improving the quality of care by identifying and eliminating defects. In respiratory care, this might include defects in clinical procedures, patient care processes, or equipment failure.

Key Six Sigma Tools in Respiratory Therapy:

- Define, Measure, Analyze, Improve, and Control (DMAIC): This is the fundamental Six Sigma process used to identify problems, measure their impact, analyze data, improve processes, and establish controls to maintain improvements.
- Control Charts: Control charts track the variation in process performance, such as response time for respiratory therapists or patient satisfaction scores, helping teams detect when performance deviates from the norm.
- Root Cause Analysis: Identifying the root cause of issues, such as high readmission rates for patients with respiratory issues, is critical for designing solutions to prevent recurrence.

4. Combining Lean and Six Sigma in Respiratory Care

The combination of Lean and Six Sigma, often referred to as Lean Six Sigma, offers a comprehensive approach to process improvement. Lean focuses on streamlining operations, while Six Sigma emphasizes reducing variation and errors. Together, they help healthcare providers deliver higher-quality, more efficient care.

For example, in a respiratory care department:

- Lean might streamline patient intake and assessment processes to reduce wait times.
- Six Sigma could be used to reduce variability in the time it takes to administer treatments or perform diagnostic tests.

By incorporating both methodologies, respiratory therapy departments can optimize both the efficiency and the quality of their care.

CREATING A CONTINUOUS IMPROVEMENT MINDSET

A continuous improvement mindset involves fostering a culture where everyone in the department is constantly looking for ways to improve their work processes, patient outcomes, and overall care delivery. It is about ensuring that quality improvement (QI) is an ongoing, never-ending process, driven by data, collaboration, and accountability.

1. Cultivating a Culture of Continuous Improvement

Creating a continuous improvement culture involves several key components:

- Leadership Commitment: Leaders must set the tone for continuous improvement by providing resources, training, and support for staff to pursue improvement initiatives.

- Staff Involvement: All team members, from respiratory therapists to support staff, should be involved in improvement efforts. Engaging staff in decision-making and problem-solving can lead to innovative solutions and buy-in for change.
- Data-Driven Decision Making: Continuous improvement relies on data to identify problems, measure progress, and make informed decisions about improvements. KPIs and other performance metrics should be used to track progress and inform decisions.
- Training and Education: Providing training on improvement methodologies like Lean, Six Sigma, and root cause analysis ensures that all staff members are equipped with the tools and knowledge to contribute to improvement efforts.
- Celebrating Successes: Recognizing and celebrating improvements, no matter how small, motivates staff and reinforces the value of continuous improvement.

2. Sustaining a Continuous Improvement Mindset

To sustain a continuous improvement mindset, respiratory therapy departments should:

- Establish Regular Review Cycles: Regularly review KPIs and improvement projects to assess progress, share results, and make adjustments where necessary.
- Encourage Experimentation: Encourage staff to try new approaches and experiment with different processes. Foster an environment where failure is seen as a learning opportunity rather than a setback.
- Create Feedback Loops: Feedback from patients, staff, and data should be continuously collected and used to refine and improve processes.

Quality improvement and evidence-based practice are essential for ensuring that respiratory care departments provide the highest level of care to their patients. KPIs help departments monitor performance, Lean and Six Sigma methodologies provide frameworks for improving efficiency and reducing errors, and a continuous improvement mindset fosters ongoing growth and progress. By focusing on these principles, respiratory therapy leaders can drive positive change in their departments, ensuring that they meet the ever-growing demands of patient care while maintaining high standards of quality.

DISCUSSION QUESTIONS

- How can respiratory therapy departments effectively integrate Lean and Six Sigma methodologies to improve patient care and operational efficiency?
- In what ways can you create a continuous improvement culture within your respiratory therapy team, and how can you ensure staff are motivated to contribute to these efforts?

MODULE NINE

LEADING INTERDISCIPLINARY TEAMS

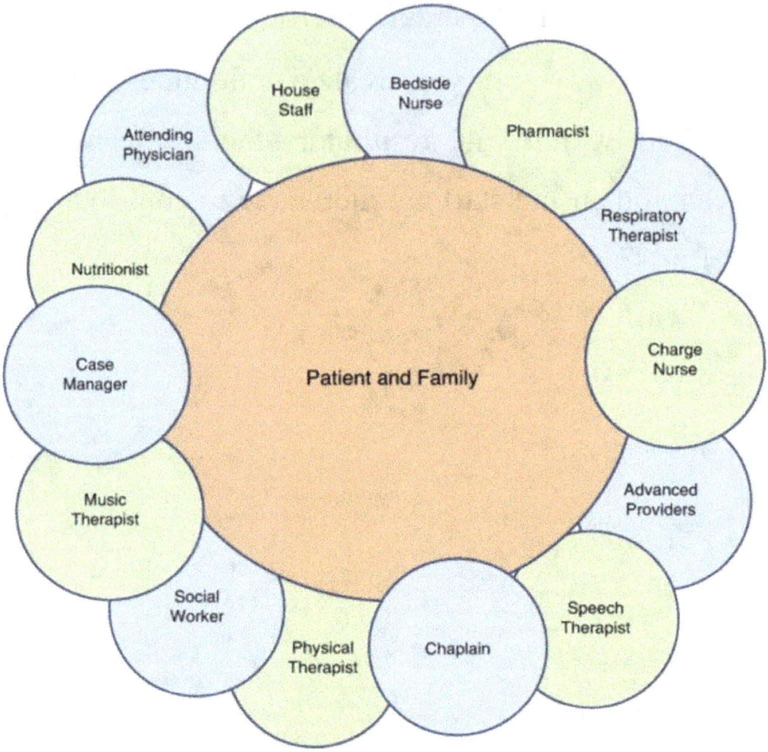

In healthcare, the most effective patient care is often the result of collaboration among various disciplines. As a respiratory leader, your role extends beyond the respiratory therapy department, requiring you to work closely with nurses, physicians, administrators, and other healthcare professionals. Leading interdisciplinary teams involves not only managing individuals from various specialties but also fostering an environment of cooperation, mutual respect, and shared goals. This module will explore how to lead interdisciplinary teams effectively, focusing on collaborating with nursing, physicians, and administration, role modeling professionalism, and managing up and across.

COLLABORATING WITH NURSING, PHYSICIANS, AND ADMINISTRATION

1. Building Effective Interdisciplinary Collaboration

Effective collaboration between respiratory therapists and other healthcare professionals is essential for delivering high-quality, patient-centered care. Respiratory therapists often work alongside nurses, physicians, and administrators to manage patients with respiratory illnesses, as well as to provide education, care plans, and assessments.

Nursing

Nurses are integral members of the healthcare team and often have firsthand knowledge of the patient's condition. Respiratory therapists must collaborate closely with nurses to:

- Coordinate care: Nurses are responsible for administering medications and monitoring patients' vital signs, while respiratory therapists manage respiratory treatments, such as nebulizer therapy or mechanical ventilation. Working together ensures that both sets of care needs are met seamlessly.

- Exchange patient information: Open communication between respiratory therapists and nurses ensures that both disciplines are aware of patient progress, reactions to treatments, and any changes in conditions.
- Provide education: Respiratory therapists can assist nurses by educating them on new respiratory treatment modalities and techniques to improve patient outcomes.

Physicians

Physicians, especially pulmonologists and critical care doctors, often drive treatment plans for patients with respiratory issues. Building a positive, collaborative relationship with physicians is crucial for ensuring optimal patient care. Respiratory leaders must:

- Understand and respect their expertise: Physicians bring a wealth of clinical knowledge, and respiratory leaders should recognize their role in diagnosing and directing treatment for respiratory conditions.
- Engage in shared decision-making: Collaborative discussions about patient diagnoses and treatment plans help ensure the best possible outcome for patients.

- Communicate effectively: Clear communication is key in addressing the needs of patients. Respiratory therapists should be able to articulate their concerns, share findings from respiratory assessments, and provide recommendations to physicians in a professional, concise manner.

Administration

In addition to collaborating with clinical teams, respiratory leaders must engage with hospital or healthcare system administration. Collaboration with administrators helps:

- Align departmental goals with hospital-wide objectives: Respiratory leaders need to ensure their department's goals align with the larger strategic vision of the healthcare organization, whether it's improving patient outcomes, reducing costs, or enhancing operational efficiency.
- Secure resources and support: Administrators are responsible for allocating budgets, staffing resources, and ensuring that the department has the necessary tools and technology to deliver optimal care. Strong relationships with administration help secure the necessary support.
- Advocate for the department: Respiratory leaders must be effective advocates for their department, communicating

its needs and successes to administrators, thus ensuring continued support for programs and initiatives.

2. Overcoming Challenges in Interdisciplinary Collaboration

Interdisciplinary collaboration is not without challenges. Respiratory leaders may encounter obstacles such as communication barriers, power dynamics, or differences in professional culture. To address these challenges:

- Encourage open dialogue: Establishing regular meetings and clear channels of communication with all team members ensures that everyone has an opportunity to contribute their perspectives and voice concerns.
- Respect diverse professional backgrounds: Each member of the healthcare team brings their own expertise, and leaders must value these contributions. A culture of mutual respect and understanding fosters stronger teamwork.
- Address conflicts promptly: Conflict, whether between disciplines or individuals, can undermine teamwork. Respiratory leaders should address issues directly, mediate when necessary, and ensure that resolutions align with the best interests of the patient.

ROLE MODELING PROFESSIONALISM

1. What is Professionalism in Respiratory Care?

Professionalism is the foundation of effective leadership in healthcare. It encompasses not only clinical expertise but also how healthcare professionals interact with one another, patients, and their families. Respiratory leaders should model professionalism in all aspects of their work.

Clinical Competence

Professional respiratory leaders must ensure they maintain high clinical standards and continue to expand their knowledge of the latest respiratory care techniques. This means:

- Staying updated with new treatments and technologies.
- Participating in ongoing education and training.
- Demonstrating proficiency in all respiratory care procedures and patient assessments.

Ethical Behavior

Respiratory leaders must adhere to ethical principles, such as honesty, integrity, confidentiality, and respect for patient autonomy. Leaders should guide their teams in:

- Protecting patient privacy: Respiratory therapists have access to sensitive patient information, and they must ensure that it is handled with confidentiality.
- Providing equitable care: Every patient, regardless of background, should receive the same level of high-quality care. Respiratory leaders should foster an environment of inclusivity and fairness.

Interpersonal Skills

A key aspect of professionalism is the ability to communicate effectively with patients, families, and interdisciplinary teams. This includes:

- Active listening: Attending to others' needs and perspectives enhances understanding and helps resolve misunderstandings.
- Conflict resolution: Addressing disagreements with tact and diplomacy is crucial in maintaining a respectful work environment.
- Empathy: Healthcare is a deeply personal service, and respiratory leaders must be able to connect with both patients and team members on a human level.

2. Modeling Professionalism for the Team

As a leader, your behavior sets the tone for your team. When you model professionalism, you create an environment where staff are encouraged to do the same. Some strategies for role modeling professionalism include:

- Demonstrating accountability: Take responsibility for your actions and decisions, and be transparent with your team.
- Embodying a patient-centered approach: Consistently prioritize patient care and encourage your team to do the same.
- Being respectful and approachable: Approach interactions with kindness and a willingness to help. This fosters an atmosphere of trust and respect within the team.

MANAGING UP AND ACROSS

1. What is Managing Up?

Managing up is the practice of working to improve the relationship between you and your superiors by proactively offering assistance, communicating effectively, and anticipating their needs. As a respiratory leader, managing up involves:

- Supporting the goals of senior leadership: Understand the larger strategic priorities of the healthcare organization and align your departmental goals accordingly.
- Communicating effectively: Be clear, concise, and proactive in sharing updates with leadership, especially when it comes to challenges and successes.
- Being solution-oriented: When presenting challenges, always bring potential solutions to the table.

Why Managing Up Matters

- It enhances trust and collaboration: Senior leaders are more likely to trust and support you if you demonstrate initiative, offer solutions, and communicate effectively.
- It promotes your department's needs: By managing up, you ensure that the respiratory department's needs are well understood at higher levels, which can help secure additional resources or attention.

2. What is Managing Across?

Managing across refers to the practice of building strong, collaborative relationships with colleagues at the same level, such as fellow department leaders or interdisciplinary team members. Managing across involves:

- Fostering collaboration: Work to align departmental efforts and priorities with other teams, including nursing, physicians, and administrators.
- Building mutual respect: Cultivate strong, positive relationships with colleagues, ensuring that they feel valued and understood.
- Sharing credit: Acknowledge the contributions of others when successes are achieved, which builds goodwill and strengthens team cohesion.

Why Managing Across Matters

- It promotes teamwork: When leaders manage across effectively, they foster an environment of mutual support and cooperation.
- It improves patient care: Collaboration among departments leads to better patient care because it ensures that all aspects of a patient's needs are addressed.

Leading interdisciplinary teams requires a combination of strong communication, professionalism, and relationship-building skills. By collaborating effectively with nursing, physicians, and administration, respiratory leaders can ensure that patient care is optimized and that the respiratory therapy department contributes meaningfully to the overall goals of the healthcare organization. Role modeling professionalism sets the standard for your team, and managing up and across helps foster trust and cooperation throughout the organization.

DISCUSSION QUESTIONS

- What are some practical steps you can take to improve collaboration between respiratory therapy and other healthcare departments, such as nursing and administration?
- How can you demonstrate professionalism in your daily interactions with both your team and interdisciplinary colleagues to foster a culture of respect and excellence?

MODULE TEN

NAVIGATING DIFFICULT CONVERSATIONS

As a respiratory leader, you will inevitably encounter difficult conversations with your team, colleagues, patients, and their families. These conversations are an essential aspect of your leadership role and can significantly impact team dynamics, patient care outcomes, and the overall working environment. Being able to navigate these conversations with confidence, compassion, and clarity is crucial to fostering a healthy, productive team culture and ensuring high-quality patient care.

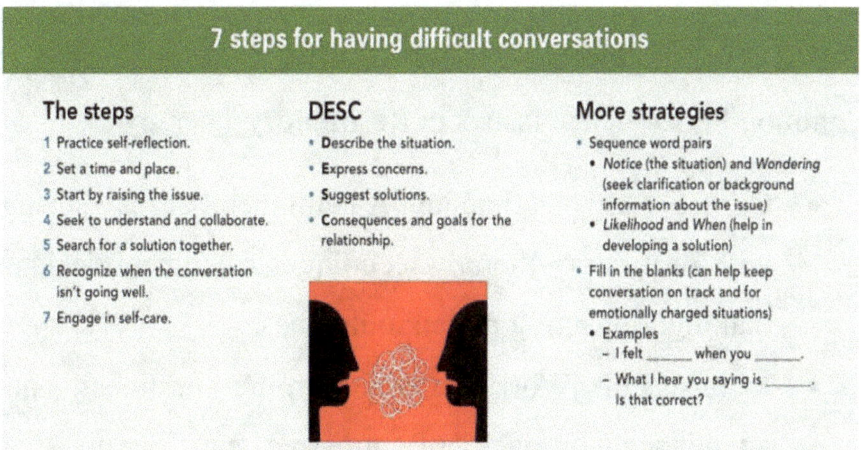

This module will explore three major areas of difficult conversations in the context of respiratory leadership: performance concerns, patient care conflicts, and cultural and generational sensitivity in team dynamics. Each of these situations requires a thoughtful, balanced approach to ensure that everyone involved feels heard, respected, and supported. Additionally, we will provide strategies and best practices to handle these conversations effectively, helping you maintain trust and respect within your team.

PERFORMANCE CONCERNS

Identifying and Addressing Performance Issues

In any healthcare environment, some team members may face performance challenges that can affect patient care and overall team morale. As a respiratory leader, it is essential to recognize when performance is not meeting expectations and address the issue in a constructive and professional manner.

Common Performance Issues in Respiratory Therapy

- Clinical Skills Deficiency: A team member may struggle with respiratory therapy techniques or clinical decision-making, impacting patient outcomes.
- Inconsistent Work Ethic: Chronic tardiness, poor attendance, or lack of initiative can disrupt team dynamics and hinder department performance.
- Lack of Teamwork: Not contributing to team goals, avoiding collaboration, or creating friction within the

group can affect the overall functioning of the department.

- Negative Attitude or Behavior: A team member's unprofessional behavior, such as hostility or resistance to feedback, can disrupt team morale and productivity.

Steps to Address Performance Concerns

- Documentation: Before having a conversation, make sure you have documented specific instances of performance concerns. Be objective and use factual examples to illustrate the issue.
- Private, Respectful Discussion: Address the performance issue privately with the individual, ensuring that you focus on the behavior rather than the person. Use "I" statements to avoid sounding accusatory (e.g., "I've noticed that you've been struggling with X task" rather than "You are always making mistakes").
- Provide Constructive Feedback: Frame your feedback in a way that highlights areas for improvement while offering support and actionable solutions. For example, if a team member is struggling with technical skills, suggest additional training or mentorship to help them grow.
- Set Clear Expectations: Ensure that the individual understands what is expected in terms of performance. Be

specific about the standards and how their work contributes to the team's success.

- Follow-up: Set a time for a follow-up meeting to monitor progress. Offer continued support and guidance to help the individual succeed.

Handling Difficult Performance Conversations

- Difficult performance conversations can be emotionally charged, especially if the individual feels defensive or attacked. To manage these situations:
- Stay Calm and Empathetic: Approach the conversation with empathy. Acknowledge any personal challenges the team member may be facing and express understanding.
- Be Solution-Oriented: Rather than focusing solely on the problem, work with the individual to come up with a plan for improvement. Highlight their strengths and how they can apply those to overcome their challenges.
- Be Patient: Changing performance patterns takes time. Provide regular feedback and celebrate small successes to maintain motivation.

PATIENT CARE CONFLICTS

Conflict Between Team Members Over Patient Care

In healthcare, conflicting opinions about patient care can arise, particularly in high-pressure situations like critical care environments. Respiratory therapists, nurses, physicians, and other healthcare providers may have differing views on the best course of action for a patient.

Common Causes of Patient Care Conflicts

- Divergent Clinical Opinions: Healthcare providers may disagree on diagnoses, treatment protocols, or the use of specific interventions for a patient.
- Differences in Priorities: Different team members may prioritize patient care in different ways, depending on their training or perspective. For example, a respiratory therapist might prioritize oxygen therapy, while a nurse might focus on pain management.
- Communication Breakdowns: Misunderstandings or lack of clear communication can lead to confusion and conflicts over the direction of care.
- Resource Allocation: Limited resources, such as equipment or time, can lead to difficult decisions that may not align with everyone's preferred course of action.

How to Address Patient Care Conflicts

Encourage Open Communication: Facilitate open dialogue where all team members can express their perspectives and concerns about the patient's care. Be sure to listen actively and validate each person's opinion.

- Focus on Patient-Centered Care: Remind the team that the ultimate goal is to provide the best possible care for the patient. Encourage the group to focus on what will most benefit the patient and resolve any disagreements with that goal in mind.
- Seek Consensus: In situations where the team cannot reach an agreement, encourage the team to find a middle ground that considers the needs of the patient and the expertise of the team. If necessary, involve a physician or another senior clinician to make the final decision.
- Respect Professional Roles: Acknowledge that each team member has a unique and important role in patient care. Respect each other's expertise and make decisions collaboratively, leveraging everyone's knowledge.

Preventing Patient Care Conflicts

- Foster a Culture of Respect: Encourage mutual respect and understanding among team members to create an environment where conflicts can be addressed constructively.

- Establish Clear Protocols: Implement clear clinical protocols and guidelines to ensure that everyone is on the same page regarding patient care. This can reduce the likelihood of disagreements about the best course of action.
- Provide Ongoing Education: Regular training and team-building activities can help healthcare providers stay aligned in their approach to patient care and reduce conflicts.

CULTURAL AND GENERATIONAL SENSITIVITY IN TEAM DYNAMICS

Understanding the Impact of Culture and Generational Differences

Healthcare teams are increasingly diverse, with individuals from different cultural backgrounds and multiple generations working together. As a respiratory leader, it's important to recognize and address the challenges that these differences may present.

Cultural Sensitivity

Cultural sensitivity involves understanding and respecting the diverse backgrounds of team members, including their customs, communication styles, and values. In a healthcare setting, cultural sensitivity is essential for:

- Fostering Inclusion: Making sure that all team members feel valued and included, regardless of their cultural background.
- Effective Communication: Being aware of language barriers, non-verbal cues, and cultural differences in communication styles can help avoid misunderstandings.
- Providing Culturally Competent Care: Understanding the cultural values and preferences of patients can enhance the quality of care provided to them.

Generational Sensitivity

Generational differences can also affect team dynamics. Each generation brings unique values, work habits, and communication preferences. The five main generations in the workforce today are:

- Traditionalists (born before 1946)
- Baby Boomers (1946-1964)
- Generation X (1965-1980)
- Millennials (1981-1996)
- Generation Z (1997-present)

Challenges of Generational Differences

Communication Styles: Older generations may prefer formal communication, while younger generations may value more informal, immediate forms of communication (e.g., texts or instant messaging).

- Work Ethics and Values: Baby Boomers may place high importance on loyalty and long-term commitment, while Millennials may prioritize work-life balance and flexibility.
- Technological Proficiency: Older generations may feel less comfortable with technology, while younger generations are typically more tech-savvy.

How to Navigate Cultural and Generational Sensitivity

- Promote Intergenerational Collaboration: Encourage team members to learn from one another and leverage the strengths of each generation. For example, older staff members may mentor younger team members, while younger staff can assist with technological tools.
- Foster an Inclusive Environment: Create a workplace culture where differences are celebrated, and all team members feel respected, regardless of their cultural or generational background.
- Provide Training on Diversity: Offer cultural competency training and workshops on generational

differences to help staff understand each other's perspectives and improve communication.

Navigating difficult conversations is an essential skill for respiratory leaders. Whether addressing performance concerns, resolving patient care conflicts, or managing cultural and generational differences, effective communication and empathy are key to maintaining a positive and productive team environment. By approaching these conversations with a solutions-oriented mindset and prioritizing mutual respect, you can foster an environment where both your team and patients thrive.

DISCUSSION QUESTIONS

- How can respiratory leaders proactively create a culture that minimizes performance concerns and supports staff development?
- What strategies can be used to address conflicts in patient care while maintaining a focus on patient-centered outcomes?

MODULE ELEVEN

LEADING THROUGH CHANGE

In healthcare, change is inevitable. From evolving clinical practices to the introduction of new technologies, regulations, and unexpected crises like pandemics, respiratory leaders must be prepared to guide their teams through periods of transition. Leading through change, particularly in clinical settings, requires adaptability, clear communication, and the ability to inspire and motivate others, even in the face of uncertainty.

- Pay attention
  - Make eye contact
  - Observe body language (theirs)
  - Remove distractions
- Show that you are listening
  - Your body language
  - Encouraging comments
- Provide feedback
  - Reflective statements
  - Clarify points
- Defer judgment
  - Listen to the "whole story"
  - Don't interrupt
- Respond appropriately
  - Be candid in your response

This module will explore three major aspects of leading through change: change management in clinical settings, leading during crises, such as the COVID-19 response, and building resilient teams that can thrive in times of change. By developing strategies to manage change effectively, respiratory leaders can not only navigate challenges but also drive improvements that benefit both staff and patients.

CHANGE MANAGEMENT IN CLINICAL SETTINGS

Change management refers to the process of preparing, supporting, and helping individuals, teams, and organizations transition from their current state to a desired future state. In clinical settings, this may include introducing new equipment, changing workflows, updating policies, or transitioning to new treatment protocols.

Why Change Management is Essential in Healthcare

Healthcare is a dynamic field. Advances in medical technology, evolving patient care standards, and healthcare reforms require healthcare professionals to constantly adapt. When a change is introduced without proper management, it can lead to confusion, resistance, and even errors that affect patient safety and care quality.

Effective change management is critical for the following reasons:

- Improved Patient Care: Implementing new clinical practices or technology can lead to better outcomes when properly managed.
- Team Engagement: When change is communicated clearly and team members are involved in the process, they are more likely to engage positively with the change.
- Reduced Resistance: Resistance to change is natural but can be mitigated with proper preparation and support.

The Process of Change Management

- Planning and Preparation: Successful change begins with understanding why the change is necessary. Involve key stakeholders early in the planning phase to understand their concerns and insights. Develop a clear roadmap for the change process.
- Communication: Communication is the cornerstone of effective change management. Ensure that all staff members understand the change, why it is happening, and what their role will be in the transition. Open channels for feedback to address any concerns.
- Training and Education: Provide adequate training to ensure that everyone feels competent and confident in

applying new protocols, technologies, or practices. This reduces anxiety and promotes smooth integration.

- Support and Reinforcement: Change can be difficult, so providing ongoing support is essential. Establish resources such as help desks, additional training sessions, and a peer support network.
- Monitoring and Feedback: Track the progress of the change and gather feedback. Evaluate what is working well and what needs to be adjusted. Be open to tweaking the approach if necessary.
- Sustaining Change: After the change has been implemented, continue reinforcing it. This could be done through regular check-ins, performance reviews, or continued education to ensure the change becomes ingrained in the team's workflow.

Overcoming Barriers to Change

In clinical settings, resistance to change is common. It can stem from:

- Fear of the Unknown: Employees may feel apprehensive about how the change will impact their roles.
- Lack of Understanding: If the reasoning behind the change is not communicated effectively, people may resist simply because they don't understand the benefits.

- Loss of Control: Change can make staff feel like they have less control over their work environment or tasks.

To overcome these barriers, respiratory leaders must build trust, provide clear information, and involve staff in the process of change.

LEADING DURING CRISIS (E.G., COVID-19 RESPONSE)

Healthcare crises, such as the COVID-19 pandemic, present unique leadership challenges. A respiratory leader's role during a crisis is not only to manage the practical aspects of care but also to support their team emotionally and mentally as they face high stress, uncertainty, and often overwhelming workloads.

Managing Clinical Operations During a Crisis

In times of crisis, the healthcare system may be overwhelmed, and leadership becomes crucial in maintaining order and ensuring continuity of care. The following strategies can help:

- Rapid Decision Making: Leaders must be able to make quick, informed decisions, often with limited information. This requires a deep understanding of clinical practice, resource availability, and the broader healthcare landscape.

- Resource Allocation: During a crisis, resources such as staff, equipment, and time may be scarce. Respiratory leaders must prioritize critical patient care needs and allocate resources efficiently.
- Adapting Protocols: Clinical guidelines and treatment protocols may change rapidly in response to new information. It is important to remain flexible and adapt to new best practices quickly.

Supporting Your Team During a Crisis

Beyond the operational aspects, leaders must also address the emotional and psychological needs of their team. Healthcare workers in crisis situations are at increased risk for burnout, anxiety, and depression. The following leadership strategies can help support them:

- Clear Communication: Communicate often and transparently with your team. Provide updates on the situation, reassure them about the changes, and explain the rationale behind decisions.
- Emotional Support: Acknowledge the stress and emotional toll that the crisis is taking on staff. Provide avenues for mental health support, such as counseling, peer support groups, and stress management resources.

- Recognition and Motivation: Crisis situations can lead to burnout if staff feel unappreciated. Regularly recognize and appreciate your team's hard work, offering both formal and informal recognition.
- Ensure Safety: Ensure that your team has access to the protective equipment and resources needed to work safely and confidently. When staff feel physically safe, they can focus better on patient care.

Lessons from the COVID-19 Response

The COVID-19 pandemic provided many lessons on how to lead during times of crisis. Respiratory leaders, in particular, were on the front lines, ensuring patients received the appropriate respiratory care, including ventilation support, oxygen therapy, and other vital treatments.

Some lessons include:

- Be Prepared for the Unexpected: While no one could predict the exact nature of the COVID-19 pandemic, being prepared with contingency plans for surges in patient volume, staffing shortages, and resource constraints is vital.
- Adapt Quickly: The ability to quickly adapt clinical and administrative workflows in response to new information is critical.

- Provide Strong Leadership Under Pressure: In times of crisis, your calm demeanor, ability to make decisions under pressure, and focus on patient care can help reassure your team and maintain morale.

BUILDING RESILIENT TEAMS

Building a resilient team is an ongoing process that pays off especially during times of change or crisis. A resilient team is able to adapt, bounce back from setbacks, and continue to deliver high-quality care even under challenging circumstances.

Key Characteristics of Resilient Teams

Strong Communication: Team members in resilient teams are not afraid to speak up, share concerns, or ask for help. They communicate openly and honestly, which fosters a culture of mutual support.

- Trust: Resilient teams have a high level of trust in each other and their leader. Team members know that they can rely on one another, and that their leader will support them.
- Flexibility: Resilient teams can quickly adjust to new information or changes. They are comfortable with ambiguity and can navigate challenges without becoming overwhelmed.

- Optimism: Resilient teams maintain a positive outlook, even in difficult times. They focus on solutions rather than problems and believe in their ability to overcome challenges.

How to Build Resilience in Your Team

- Provide Training and Development: Build resilience through continuous learning and professional development. Equip your team with the skills they need to handle new challenges and changes in healthcare.
- Foster a Supportive Environment: Create a work environment where team members feel valued and supported. Encourage collaboration, celebrate successes, and provide constructive feedback.
- Encourage Work-Life Balance: Resilience is not just about handling stress at work but also about ensuring that your team members have time to recharge. Encourage regular breaks, time off, and self-care.
- Promote a Growth Mindset: Encourage your team to view challenges as opportunities for growth. A growth mindset helps individuals and teams stay focused on improvement and overcoming adversity.

Building Resilient Teams Through Crisis

A key component of leading through change is ensuring that your team can manage and bounce back from crisis situations. Building resilience means preparing them not only to handle the immediate pressure of a crisis but also to learn from it and emerge stronger.

Leading through change requires a comprehensive understanding of change management, crisis leadership, and team resilience. As a respiratory leader, it is essential to remain adaptable, communicate effectively, and provide support to your team. Whether you are navigating the introduction of a new clinical practice or leading your team through a healthcare crisis like COVID-19, resilience, clear communication, and strong leadership are the foundations of success.

By fostering a resilient team that can adapt to change and manage challenges effectively, you will create an environment where both staff and patients thrive, even in the most difficult times.

DISCUSSION QUESTIONS

- What strategies can respiratory leaders use to build a resilient team that is prepared for unforeseen crises?

- How can respiratory leaders balance the immediate need for crisis management with the long-term goal of creating sustainable change and improvement within their departments?

MODULE TWELVE

THE NEXT GENERATION OF RESPIRATORY LEADERS

The future of respiratory care depends not only on the development of new technologies and clinical advancements but also on the cultivation of strong, capable leaders who can guide the next generation of respiratory therapists. Respiratory leadership does not stop with the current team; it must be passed on, nurtured, and developed in those who will take on leadership roles in the future. This module focuses on the essential components of preparing and developing the next generation of respiratory leaders, including succession planning, fostering leadership in bedside therapists, and developing a legacy of excellence.

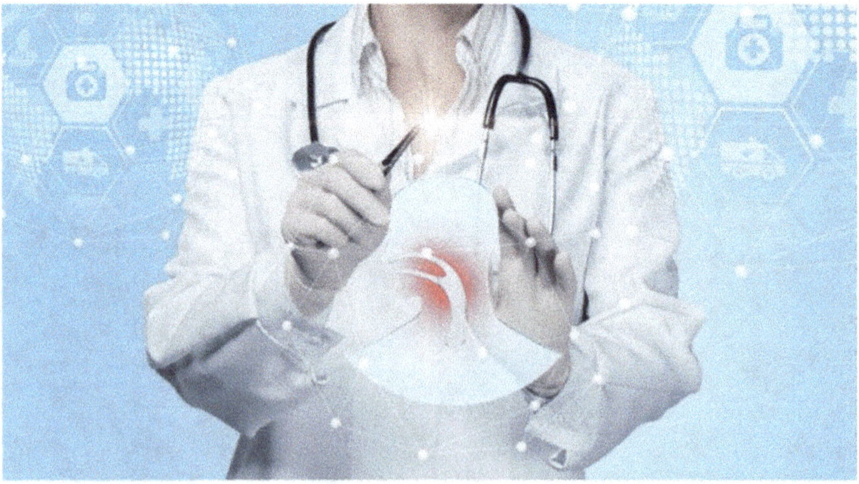

SUCCESSION PLANNING

Succession planning is the process of identifying and developing future leaders within an organization to ensure the continued success and sustainability of the department or organization. In respiratory care, effective succession planning is critical as it ensures that there are qualified individuals ready to step into leadership roles when current leaders retire, move on, or transition into other roles.

Why Succession Planning Matters in Respiratory Care

Respiratory therapy departments, like many healthcare organizations, are facing a wave of retirements and an increasing demand for leadership. Without a clear succession plan, departments may experience gaps in leadership, leading to a loss of knowledge, decreased morale, and potential disruptions in patient care.

Effective succession planning helps to:

- Ensure Continuity: By identifying potential leaders early on, departments can ensure a smooth transition when senior leaders move on or retire.
- Develop Talent: Succession planning is not just about filling vacancies but also about nurturing and developing

the leadership potential of employees who are committed to advancing their careers.

- Enhance Departmental Stability: When leadership is handed over to well-prepared individuals, the department remains stable, and transitions happen with minimal disruption.

Key Steps in Succession Planning

- Identify Critical Roles: Start by identifying which roles within the department will need to be filled in the future. For respiratory therapy, this could include supervisory roles, department heads, or clinical coordinators.
- Assess Current and Future Needs: Consider the department's future needs. What will the role of a respiratory leader look like in five to ten years? What skills, knowledge, and competencies will be required to succeed in that role?
- Talent Identification: Look at current team members who demonstrate leadership potential. These individuals may show a combination of strong clinical skills, emotional intelligence, and a desire for career advancement.
- Develop a Leadership Pipeline: Once potential leaders are identified, invest in their development. Offer training,

mentorship, and opportunities to take on leadership responsibilities in a supportive environment.

- Provide Ongoing Development: Even after an individual has been identified for a leadership role, provide continuous development. This could include leadership workshops, exposure to management tasks, and opportunities for networking.
- Evaluate and Adjust: Regularly review your succession planning strategy. Leadership needs and organizational goals can shift, so ensure that your succession plan stays aligned with departmental and institutional priorities.

Challenges of Succession Planning

While succession planning is essential, it can present challenges, such as:

- Resistance to Change: Established leaders may be reluctant to pass on the reins, creating resistance to succession planning. Overcoming this requires a clear vision for the department's future and a willingness to develop others.
- Limited Resources: Small departments may not have the resources to invest in leadership development. Creative solutions such as mentorship programs or shared leadership responsibilities can mitigate this challenge.

- Succession Gaps: There may be a lack of qualified candidates to step into leadership positions, especially if the current generation of leaders has not focused on mentoring younger staff. To address this, departments must prioritize leadership development from an early stage.

FOSTERING LEADERSHIP IN BEDSIDE THERAPISTS

Bedside respiratory therapists are at the heart of patient care, and many of them possess valuable leadership qualities that can be harnessed to improve both patient outcomes and team dynamics. Fostering leadership in bedside therapists involves identifying opportunities for them to take on leadership roles, even before they step into formal management positions.

Why Fostering Leadership in Bedside Therapists is Critical

Bedside therapists interact directly with patients and have invaluable insight into the day-to-day operations of the respiratory care department. They possess strong clinical expertise, critical thinking skills, and the ability to manage high-pressure situations. These qualities make them ideal candidates for leadership roles, yet many therapists do not initially see themselves as leaders.

Fostering leadership at the bedside helps to:

- Enhance Patient Care: Therapists who take on leadership roles can positively impact patient care by improving workflows, optimizing clinical practices, and encouraging team collaboration.
- Empower Therapists: Providing leadership opportunities empowers bedside therapists to take ownership of their work, leading to greater job satisfaction, engagement, and retention.
- Bridge the Gap Between Frontline Care and Leadership: Bedside therapists who are groomed for leadership positions understand the challenges faced by frontline workers, which makes them effective leaders who can drive change while maintaining high clinical standards.

How to Foster Leadership in Bedside Therapists

- Provide Leadership Development Opportunities: Leadership development for bedside therapists should not be limited to formal management training. Encourage informal leadership opportunities by giving therapists the chance to mentor new staff, lead patient care initiatives, or take part in quality improvement projects.
- Encourage Autonomy and Decision-Making: Give bedside therapists the autonomy to make decisions within

their scope of practice. Trusting them to take charge of patient care decisions fosters their confidence and leadership abilities.

- Mentorship and Coaching: Pair experienced leaders with bedside therapists to provide mentorship and coaching. This will allow them to learn the nuances of leadership, communication, and decision-making from those who have experience.
- Recognize Leadership Contributions: Recognizing leadership in any form can have a significant impact. Celebrate therapists who take initiative, lead quality improvement projects, or demonstrate leadership in patient care situations.
- Create Opportunities for Peer Leadership: Leadership isn't always about managing people. Encourage bedside therapists to take on leadership roles in guiding their peers, solving problems collaboratively, or contributing to team education.

DEVELOPING A LEGACY OF EXCELLENCE

A legacy of excellence goes beyond achieving short-term goals; it's about creating a culture that consistently prioritizes high standards, continuous improvement, and ethical practices. For respiratory leaders, developing a legacy of excellence means leaving a long-lasting impact on the department, fostering a culture where future leaders can thrive, and ensuring that patient care remains at the highest standard.

The Importance of a Legacy of Excellence

Developing a legacy of excellence in respiratory care is about more than simply meeting current standards; it's about creating a foundation for sustained success. A strong legacy inspires future leaders and sets the bar for the quality of care delivered by the department, even in the face of challenges. This legacy shapes not only clinical outcomes but also the environment in which clinicians and patients interact.

Building a Legacy of Excellence

Foster a Culture of Continuous Improvement: Excellence is an ongoing pursuit. Leaders should encourage ongoing professional development, innovation, and participation in quality improvement initiatives. By embedding a culture of continuous improvement, respiratory leaders ensure that the department's performance will only get better over time.

- Establish Clear Standards and Expectations: Set clear expectations for both clinical practice and professional conduct. Leaders should communicate high standards and ensure that these are upheld consistently across all levels of the team.

- Lead by Example: Leaders must model the behavior and attitudes they wish to see in others. This includes demonstrating professionalism, a commitment to high-quality care, and an openness to feedback and growth.
- Invest in the Development of Future Leaders: As discussed in earlier sections, investing in the next generation of respiratory leaders is crucial for building a lasting legacy. Leaders should identify and mentor rising stars within the department, providing them with the skills and guidance needed to carry the department forward.
- Celebrate Successes and Learn from Failures: Recognize achievements and use them as opportunities to reinforce the importance of quality care. When things don't go as planned, take time to reflect, learn from the experience, and incorporate the lessons into future practices.

Leaving a Legacy Through Influence

A legacy is often a product of influence, not authority. By influencing your team to adopt a mindset of excellence, leaders ensure that the standards of care, professionalism, and patient advocacy continue long after they leave. The legacy of a respiratory leader is reflected in the work of their successors and the culture they help to shape.

Succession planning, fostering leadership in bedside therapists, and developing a legacy of excellence are essential components in preparing the next generation of respiratory leaders. By developing future leaders and creating a culture that prioritizes high standards and continuous improvement, respiratory departments can ensure a bright future for their staff and the patients they serve.

A strong, forward-thinking leadership strategy will provide the framework for success, even as the landscape of healthcare continues to evolve.

DISCUSSION QUESTIONS

- What are some strategies that respiratory leaders can implement to identify and develop leadership potential in their team members, especially those in bedside therapy roles?
- How can a legacy of excellence in a respiratory department be sustained beyond the tenure of current leaders, and how can the next generation be empowered to continue this tradition?

MODULE THIRTEEN

THE CALL TO LEAD IN RESPIRATORY CARE

In the dynamic and ever-evolving field of healthcare, leadership within respiratory therapy (RT) plays a crucial role in ensuring not only the effective delivery of clinical care but also the development of a team culture that fosters innovation, collaboration, and quality. This module explores the foundational aspects of leadership in respiratory care, from understanding why leadership matters to defining what excellence in clinical care and team culture entails, and how professionals can evolve from clinicians to agents of change.

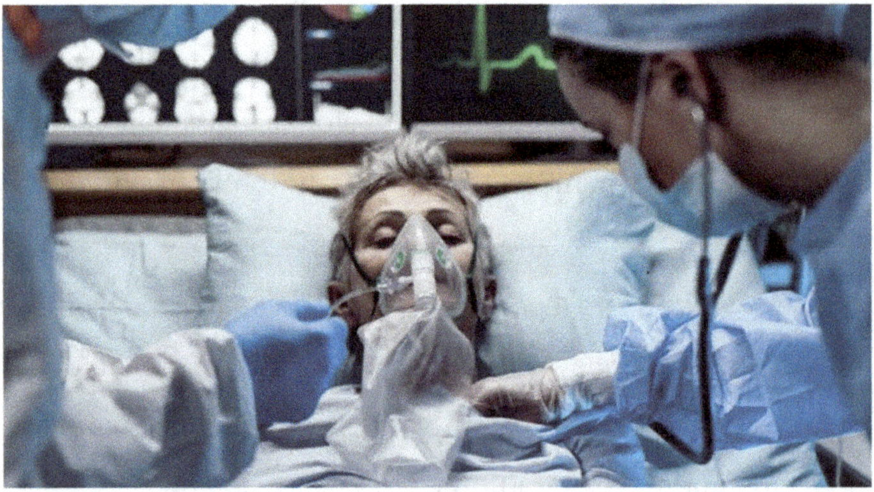

WHY LEADERSHIP MATTERS IN RESPIRATORY THERAPY

Respiratory therapy is a vital component of modern healthcare, addressing the prevention, diagnosis, and treatment of respiratory conditions. Respiratory therapists (RTs) provide critical care across various settings, from emergency rooms and intensive care units (ICUs) to outpatient clinics and home care. They work in interdisciplinary teams with physicians, nurses, and other healthcare professionals, collaborating to ensure the best outcomes for patients with respiratory issues such as asthma, chronic obstructive pulmonary disease (COPD), and pneumonia.

However, respiratory therapy is not only about direct patient care. The need for leadership within this field is paramount. Effective leadership in respiratory care ensures that clinical practices are evidence-based, that resources are optimized, and that teams work harmoniously toward common goals. The leadership skills of an RT leader are as crucial as their clinical expertise, as they are responsible for setting the tone of the department, advocating for their team members, and spearheading innovations in patient care.

Why Leadership is Crucial in Respiratory Therapy

- Advancing Clinical Care Standards: Respiratory care is constantly evolving with advances in technology, pharmaceuticals, and clinical practices. Leadership helps ensure that respiratory teams stay ahead of the curve by implementing new techniques, staying informed on best practices, and adapting to emerging trends. Without strong leadership, departments may become complacent, and patient care could suffer.
- Improving Patient Outcomes: Effective leadership in respiratory therapy directly impacts patient outcomes. When leaders guide their teams to provide high-quality care, set clear expectations, and encourage a patient-centered approach, the results speak for themselves. Studies show that high-quality leadership leads to better team communication, which in turn results in fewer errors and improved patient safety.
- Resource Optimization and Efficiency: Leaders in respiratory therapy departments are responsible for managing the resources at their disposal, including staff, equipment, and financial resources. Good leadership ensures that these resources are used effectively, reducing waste and ensuring the smooth running of the department. For example, a leader may streamline

processes for equipment use, ensuring that the department runs efficiently while still meeting the needs of patients.

- Team Morale and Cohesion: Leadership plays a significant role in team dynamics. When respiratory care leaders promote collaboration, trust, and open communication, it fosters an environment where team members feel valued and supported. This leads to higher job satisfaction, better retention rates, and a more cohesive team that works well together under pressure.
- Adaptation to Changes in Healthcare: Healthcare is a constantly changing landscape, with new regulations, technologies, and patient needs emerging regularly. Respiratory therapy leaders must be equipped to adapt to these changes, advocating for their teams, ensuring compliance with new standards, and implementing strategies that keep their departments at the forefront of care delivery.

DEFINING EXCELLENCE IN CLINICAL CARE AND TEAM CULTURE

Leadership in respiratory therapy is not just about guiding clinical practice; it is about defining and maintaining a culture of excellence in care and team performance. Excellence is the foundation on which effective respiratory leadership is built. A commitment to excellence requires clear standards, continuous evaluation, and a focus on both individual and team growth.

Defining Excellence in Clinical Care

Excellence in clinical care in respiratory therapy means providing the highest standard of care to patients, tailored to their individual needs and guided by evidence-based practices. It involves a commitment to improving patient outcomes by applying the latest research, technologies, and methodologies while maintaining a patient-centered approach.

Key elements of clinical excellence in respiratory care include:

- Evidence-Based Practices: Excellence requires staying informed about the latest research and applying evidence-based techniques to care. This can include the latest advancements in mechanical ventilation, airway management, and diagnostic testing.
- Patient-Centered Approach: Every patient is unique, and providing excellent respiratory care means considering the patient's individual needs, preferences, and circumstances. Leaders must ensure that their teams approach every patient with empathy, respect, and professionalism.

- Adherence to Best Practices: Leaders should establish and maintain protocols based on the best available evidence and ensure these are implemented consistently across the department. This includes training staff on proper techniques and ensuring regular audits to ensure compliance.

Building a Culture of Excellence in Team Dynamics

A culture of excellence is not limited to clinical care. It extends to how teams interact with each other, collaborate, and grow together. A strong team culture in respiratory therapy departments ensures that team members support one another, continuously improve, and are motivated to achieve both individual and collective goals.

Key components of a culture of excellence include:

- Clear Communication: Communication is the backbone of any high-performing team. Leaders must foster an environment where open, honest, and effective communication is encouraged at all levels. This ensures that everyone is on the same page, prevents misunderstandings, and enhances collaboration.
- Accountability: In a culture of excellence, everyone is held accountable for their actions and performance. Respiratory care leaders must establish clear expectations

for both individual and team performance and provide regular feedback. Accountability also involves fostering a climate where team members can give and receive constructive feedback, helping everyone improve.

- Continuous Learning and Development: Excellence in respiratory care requires a commitment to ongoing education and professional growth. Leaders must encourage and provide opportunities for staff to attend workshops, gain certifications, and participate in conferences. This commitment to learning helps ensure that the team stays at the cutting edge of respiratory care practices.
- Recognition and Motivation: Recognizing individual and team accomplishments helps to build morale and encourage continued excellence. Whether it's through formal awards, informal praise, or leadership's visible support, recognition helps individuals feel valued and motivates them to maintain high standards.

THE JOURNEY FROM CLINICIAN TO CHANGE AGENT

Respiratory therapists typically start their careers as clinicians, providing hands-on care to patients. Over time, however, many therapists are called to evolve beyond their clinical roles and take on leadership responsibilities. This journey from clinician to leader is not only about acquiring new skills and responsibilities but also about embracing a broader role as a change agent within the healthcare system.

The Shift from Clinician to Leader

The transition from clinician to leader involves a fundamental shift in mindset. As clinicians, respiratory therapists focus primarily on individual patient care, utilizing their technical expertise and clinical judgment. However, as leaders, they are responsible for much more than direct care—they must guide teams, improve departmental processes, and advocate for better patient outcomes across the board.

Key aspects of this journey include:

- Developing Leadership Skills: Respiratory therapists must develop leadership skills such as communication, problem-solving, decision-making, and emotional intelligence. These skills go beyond clinical expertise and are essential for motivating teams and driving change within the department.
- Adapting to a New Role: Leadership involves stepping back from the direct patient care role and focusing more on strategic planning, staff development, and departmental operations. This shift can be challenging, as

it requires therapists to manage resources, navigate institutional politics, and guide others to achieve common goals.

- Embracing Change: Leaders are often the drivers of change within their teams and departments. A key part of being a change agent is having the courage and vision to challenge the status quo, implement new practices, and advocate for innovations that will improve patient care and team performance.

The Role of a Change Agent

Change agents within respiratory care leadership are individuals who actively seek to transform their department or institution by improving processes, introducing new technologies, and creating a culture of excellence. As change agents, leaders are responsible for identifying areas for improvement, inspiring their teams to embrace these changes, and ensuring that the changes are successfully implemented.

Key characteristics of effective change agents include:

- Visionary Thinking: Successful leaders are visionaries who can see the bigger picture and foresee the future direction of the field. They anticipate trends in healthcare and respiratory care and position their departments to be at the forefront of these changes.

- Influencing Others: A change agent's ability to influence others is critical. This involves motivating staff to embrace new practices and ensuring that the department is aligned with the broader goals of the healthcare system.
- Resilience and Adaptability: Change often meets resistance, but effective leaders understand how to navigate these challenges. They demonstrate resilience, stay focused on their goals, and adapt their strategies as needed to ensure the change is sustainable.

DISCUSSION QUESTIONS

- What leadership traits are essential for respiratory therapists transitioning from clinical roles to leadership roles, and how can they develop these traits effectively?
- In what ways can respiratory therapy departments create a culture of excellence that fosters both clinical care quality and a strong, collaborative team environment?

MODULE FOURTEEN

CORE PRINCIPLES OF RESPIRATORY LEADERSHIP

In the field of respiratory care, strong leadership is not just about managing a department or directing clinical practices. It is about embodying core values, possessing specific competencies, and adhering to ethical standards that guide actions, decisions, and interactions with others. The most effective leaders are those who combine technical expertise with a strong ethical framework, interpersonal sensitivity, and a deep understanding of the importance of patient-centered care. This module will explore the core principles of respiratory leadership, including servant leadership, emotional intelligence, ethical decision-making, and professionalism, as these foundational elements are crucial for developing high-quality, compassionate leadership in clinical settings.

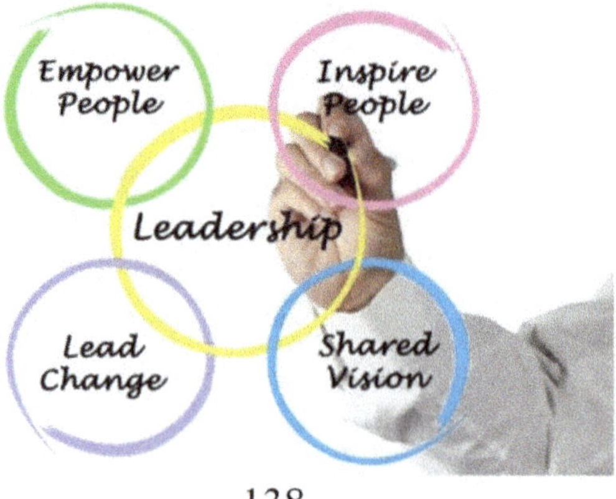

SERVANT LEADERSHIP IN CLINICAL SETTINGS

Servant leadership is a philosophy and set of practices that prioritize the growth and well-being of individuals, teams, and communities. This leadership model is particularly important in healthcare, where the focus should be on patient care and team empowerment. A servant leader does not seek personal gain or recognition; instead, they are committed to serving others, which leads to the flourishing of individuals and teams. This is particularly relevant in respiratory therapy, where team members rely heavily on each other, and a collaborative, supportive environment is necessary to provide the best patient care.

Key Characteristics of Servant Leadership in Respiratory Care

Empathy and Listening: A servant leader in respiratory care is genuinely concerned with the well-being of their team members and patients. They take the time to listen to their staff's concerns and provide support, fostering an environment where individuals feel heard and valued. In clinical settings, this translates into better patient care, as staff members are more motivated and capable of delivering high-quality, compassionate care when they feel understood and supported.

- Stewardship and Accountability: Servant leaders act as stewards of their resources, including human resources. They take responsibility for the professional growth of their team members, providing the necessary tools, training, and opportunities to advance their skills. Additionally, they hold themselves and their team accountable, ensuring that everyone adheres to best practices, institutional policies, and ethical standards in patient care.
- Commitment to the Growth of Others: Servant leadership places a strong emphasis on the development of others, not only in technical skills but also in emotional and psychological growth. Leaders who adopt this model are committed to mentoring their staff, helping them develop professionally, and supporting their personal well-being. In respiratory therapy, this involves offering ongoing education and opportunities for growth, ensuring that the team is prepared for the ever-changing healthcare environment.
- Building Community: Respiratory therapy departments often work in highly stressful environments, particularly in intensive care units or emergency settings. Servant leaders help foster a sense of community within the team, where collaboration and mutual respect are the

foundation. By creating a culture of community, leaders ensure that their teams are cohesive, able to work well under pressure, and feel supported in their roles.

Impact of Servant Leadership on Patient Care and Team Morale

Servant leadership enhances patient care by cultivating a workplace culture where the needs of both the patients and the staff are prioritized. When leaders serve their teams, team members are more likely to go above and beyond for their patients, demonstrating compassion, care, and competence. This leads to improved patient outcomes and enhanced satisfaction.

Emotional Intelligence and Self-Awareness

Emotional intelligence (EQ) is the ability to recognize, understand, and manage one's own emotions, as well as the emotions of others. In healthcare, particularly in respiratory therapy, emotional intelligence is a cornerstone of effective leadership. It allows leaders to navigate the complex emotional dynamics of clinical settings, build strong relationships with team members, and handle stressful situations with poise and insight.

Components of Emotional Intelligence for Respiratory Leaders

Self-Awareness: This is the foundation of emotional intelligence. Self-aware leaders understand their own emotions, strengths, weaknesses, and how their actions impact others. In respiratory leadership, self-awareness is crucial because it helps leaders manage their reactions, particularly in high-pressure situations, such as during patient emergencies or conflicts within the team.

- Self-Regulation: Respiratory care leaders must manage their emotions effectively, especially in stressful or challenging situations. Self-regulation allows leaders to stay calm, make thoughtful decisions, and prevent emotional reactions from clouding their judgment. It also helps to avoid conflicts or making hasty decisions that may harm the team or patient outcomes.
- Empathy: Empathy is the ability to understand and share the feelings of others. Leaders with high emotional intelligence are able to recognize the emotional state of their team members and respond appropriately. This helps to build trust and rapport with staff, ensuring that they feel supported and valued. In patient care,

empathetic leaders guide their teams to provide care that is compassionate and patient-centered.

- Social Skills: Effective communication, conflict resolution, and relationship-building are essential components of emotional intelligence. Respiratory leaders with strong social skills are able to foster collaboration, inspire their teams, and create a positive work environment. Strong social skills also enable leaders to negotiate with other healthcare professionals, ensuring that respiratory care is integrated effectively within interdisciplinary teams.
- Motivation: Leaders with high EQ are driven not just by personal goals but by a desire to achieve positive outcomes for their team and patients. This intrinsic motivation is contagious and can inspire the entire team to strive for excellence.

Impact of Emotional Intelligence on Leadership Effectiveness

Leaders with high emotional intelligence are able to build trust, resolve conflicts effectively, and inspire their teams to excel. In respiratory therapy, where patient care often requires coordination with various healthcare professionals, strong emotional intelligence enhances collaboration, reduces misunderstandings, and promotes a more cohesive team dynamic.

ETHICAL DECISION-MAKING IN RESPIRATORY PRACTICE

Ethical decision-making is essential in healthcare, where the stakes are high, and decisions can profoundly affect the lives of patients. In respiratory therapy, leaders are often called upon to make difficult ethical decisions, such as whether to initiate or discontinue life-supporting treatments, how to allocate resources during shortages, or how to balance patient autonomy with clinical guidelines.

Principles of Ethical Decision-Making in Respiratory Care

Beneficence and Non-Maleficence: Leaders in respiratory therapy must prioritize the well-being of their patients by acting in their best interests and avoiding harm. This involves making decisions that promote patient health, dignity, and comfort while minimizing unnecessary risks.

- Autonomy: Patient autonomy is a key ethical principle. Leaders must ensure that patients are informed of their options, can make their own decisions regarding their care, and are treated with respect. This can be particularly challenging in cases where patients are unable to make decisions for themselves or where there are cultural or familial pressures that conflict with clinical recommendations.

- Justice: In a healthcare setting, leaders must strive for fairness and equity in the distribution of resources and care. This principle is particularly relevant in resource-limited settings or during public health crises, where difficult choices may need to be made about who receives care and what interventions are prioritized.
- Confidentiality and Privacy: Respiratory leaders must maintain patient confidentiality and adhere to privacy laws such as HIPAA in the United States. This includes ensuring that sensitive patient information is not disclosed improperly and that patient rights are protected.
- Professional Integrity: Ethical decision-making in respiratory therapy requires leaders to be transparent, honest, and accountable for their actions. They must act with integrity, ensuring that decisions are based on sound clinical evidence, professional guidelines, and ethical standards.

Strategies for Promoting Ethical Decision-Making

Fostering an Ethical Culture: Leaders can promote an ethical culture by discussing ethical dilemmas openly with their teams, providing ethics training, and ensuring that staff have access to ethical guidance when needed.

- Interdisciplinary Collaboration: Ethical decisions in respiratory care often involve collaboration with other healthcare professionals. Leaders should foster interdisciplinary collaboration to ensure that all perspectives are considered when making ethical decisions.
- Ethics Committees: Many healthcare organizations have ethics committees that provide guidance on difficult cases. Leaders can leverage these committees to ensure that ethical decisions are made with input from a range of experts.

PROFESSIONALISM, INTEGRITY, AND TRUST

Professionalism, integrity, and trust are the cornerstones of effective leadership in respiratory therapy. These qualities are essential for building strong relationships with patients, families, and interdisciplinary teams. Respiratory leaders must model these traits to cultivate a work environment where trust is paramount, and ethical conduct is the norm.

Professionalism in Respiratory Leadership

Professionalism in respiratory therapy encompasses several components, including:

- Competence: Leaders must maintain and enhance their technical skills to provide the best possible care to patients. This requires continuous learning, attending training, and staying updated on best practices.
- Respect: Professional leaders demonstrate respect for their colleagues, patients, and families by listening actively, showing empathy, and treating others with dignity.
- Accountability: Leaders must hold themselves and their teams accountable for their actions, ensuring that everyone adheres to high standards of practice and behavior.

Integrity and Trust in Leadership

Integrity involves adhering to moral and ethical principles even when it is difficult. Leaders who act with integrity build trust among their teams, which is essential for creating a positive and productive work environment. Trust is a key component of effective leadership, and it is built over time through consistent actions that reflect honesty, fairness, and ethical decision-making.

DISCUSSION QUESTIONS

- How can respiratory leaders use emotional intelligence to improve team communication and resolve conflicts in high-pressure clinical settings?
- What steps can respiratory therapy leaders take to ensure that ethical decision-making is prioritized in their departments, and how can they foster an ethical culture within their teams?

MODULE FIFTEEN

CREATING A CULTURE OF EXCELLENCE IN RESPIRATORY LEADERSHIP

A culture of excellence is one where every team member feels motivated, trusted, and empowered to deliver their best work, ultimately enhancing patient outcomes. Achieving this requires intentional efforts to build a cohesive, high-performing team, foster open and supportive communication, ensure accountability without blame, and create a psychologically safe environment.

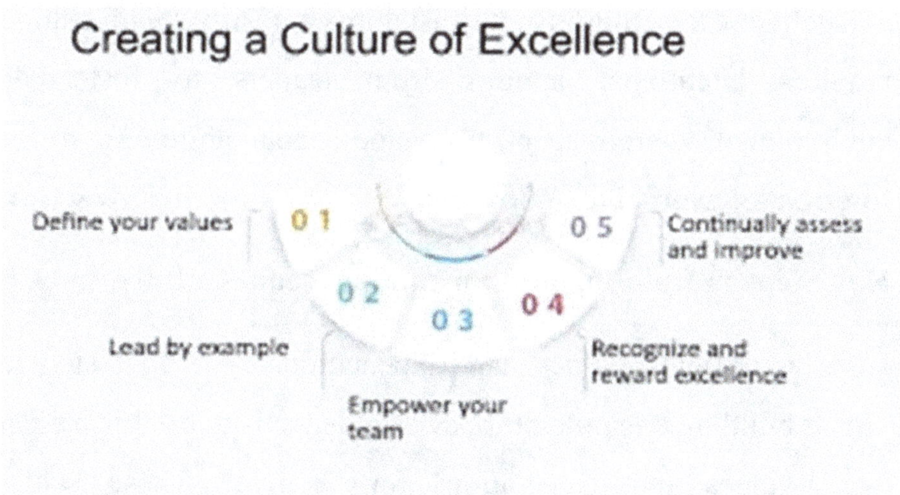

This module will explore these key components: building and sustaining team culture, motivating teams through engagement and purpose, ensuring accountability without blame, and fostering psychological safety and empowerment. These elements are crucial for creating a thriving, high-functioning respiratory therapy team that is capable of providing the best care to patients while supporting the professional growth and well-being of each team member.

BUILDING AND SUSTAINING TEAM CULTURE

A strong team culture is a vital foundation for any successful healthcare department, especially in respiratory therapy, where collaboration and trust are paramount. Culture within a team refers to the shared values, norms, and behaviors that shape how team members interact with one another, approach their work, and deliver care. Building and sustaining a positive team culture requires intentional actions from leaders to foster an environment where respect, trust, and accountability are at the forefront of every interaction.

Key Steps in Building and Sustaining Team Culture

- Clarifying Values and Expectations: The first step in building a team culture of excellence is to establish clear values and expectations for behavior. These values should align with the hospital's overall mission and vision but should also reflect the unique needs of the respiratory care department. For example, a respiratory care team might prioritize values such as empathy, integrity, innovation, teamwork, and continuous learning. Once these values are defined, they must be communicated clearly and consistently across the team.

- Role Modeling by Leadership: Leaders play a crucial role in shaping and sustaining team culture. Leaders must model the values and behaviors they wish to see in their team. For example, if collaboration is a core value, the leader must engage in collaborative decision-making, encourage input from team members, and celebrate collective achievements. Leaders who exemplify these behaviors set a strong example for others to follow, reinforcing the desired culture.
- Encouraging Open Communication: Communication is the cornerstone of a strong team culture. Leaders must foster an environment where team members feel safe and encouraged to communicate openly, ask questions, and share ideas. Regular team meetings, feedback sessions, and informal check-ins can promote transparency and encourage dialogue between team members and leadership.
- Celebrating Successes and Learning from Challenges: A strong team culture also involves recognizing and celebrating successes, both big and small. Public acknowledgment of individual and team

accomplishments boosts morale and reinforces positive behaviors. At the same time, it is important to approach challenges and failures as learning opportunities. A culture of excellence does not shy away from mistakes; instead, it views them as an opportunity to grow and improve.

- Creating Opportunities for Team Bonding: Team bonding activities help to build relationships and trust among team members. These activities can range from casual social gatherings to team-building exercises that improve collaboration and problem-solving skills. When team members feel connected on a personal level, they are more likely to collaborate effectively in a clinical setting.

Sustaining Team Culture

Sustaining a team culture of excellence requires continuous effort and reinforcement. Culture is not something that can be built once and left to grow on its own. Leaders must regularly assess the team's cultural health and make adjustments as needed. Regularly revisiting the team's values, celebrating achievements, addressing challenges, and providing feedback help keep the culture alive and evolving.

MOTIVATING TEAMS: STRATEGIES FOR ENGAGEMENT AND PURPOSE

Motivating teams, especially in a high-pressure environment like respiratory care, is one of the most important responsibilities of a leader. Motivation drives performance, engagement, and job satisfaction, and it directly impacts the quality of care provided to patients. Motivated teams are more likely to go above and beyond, remain committed to their work, and support each other through challenges.

Strategies for Engaging and Motivating Teams

- Providing Clear Purpose and Vision: A critical motivational strategy is to provide team members with a clear sense of purpose and vision. When respiratory therapists understand how their work contributes to the overall success of the healthcare system and the well-being of patients, they are more likely to feel engaged and committed. Leaders should regularly communicate the team's goals, the broader mission of the department, and the impact of their work on patient outcomes. This helps to connect day-to-day tasks with the greater purpose of patient care and hospital success.
- Recognizing Contributions: Recognition is a powerful motivator. Publicly acknowledging team members for

their hard work, dedication, and accomplishments boosts morale and reinforces desired behaviors. Leaders can create formal recognition programs or simply take time to thank individuals for their contributions during team meetings. Small gestures of appreciation, such as personalized thank-you notes or a "shout-out" during a meeting, can have a significant impact on team motivation.

- Offering Opportunities for Growth and Development: Professionals in respiratory care are motivated when they see opportunities for personal and professional growth. Leaders should invest in training, continuing education, and mentorship opportunities that allow team members to expand their knowledge and skills. Offering career advancement opportunities and a clear path for progression within the department shows employees that they are valued and that their growth matters.
- Empowering Team Members: Empowerment is a powerful motivational tool. When team members feel they have the autonomy to make decisions and take ownership of their work, they are more likely to be engaged and motivated. Leaders should encourage decision-making at all levels, provide opportunities for

input, and trust team members to make important contributions to patient care and department operations.

- Creating a Supportive Work Environment: A positive work environment is essential for motivation. Leaders should focus on creating an environment where team members feel safe, respected, and valued. This includes addressing any issues related to work-life balance, providing necessary resources and support, and encouraging healthy relationships among team members. A supportive environment fosters a sense of belonging and increases engagement.

ACCOUNTABILITY WITHOUT BLAME

Accountability is crucial in healthcare settings, where mistakes or lapses in care can have serious consequences for patient outcomes. However, accountability does not need to be synonymous with blame. Leaders must foster a culture where team members are held accountable for their actions and responsibilities, but also feel supported and encouraged to improve rather than punished for mistakes.

Building a Culture of Accountability Without Blame

- Clear Expectations: To ensure accountability, leaders must set clear expectations regarding roles, responsibilities, and performance standards. When expectations are clearly communicated and understood, team members are more likely to take ownership of their actions and outcomes. Additionally, leaders should regularly check in with team members to provide feedback, answer questions, and offer support as needed.

- Focus on Solutions, Not Punishment: When mistakes happen, leaders should focus on finding solutions rather than placing blame. This involves analyzing the situation, identifying contributing factors, and working with the team to prevent similar issues in the future. Leaders should encourage an open dialogue where team members feel safe admitting mistakes and learning from them.
- Constructive Feedback: Providing constructive feedback is a key component of accountability. Leaders should offer feedback in a way that is respectful, objective, and focused on improvement. This type of feedback helps individuals understand how they can grow and develop without feeling attacked or demeaned.
- Support for Improvement: Leaders must provide the support necessary for team members to meet expectations and improve performance. This may include additional training, mentoring, or other resources to help team members succeed. When team members know that they will be supported in their efforts to improve, they are

more likely to take responsibility for their actions and work toward better outcomes.

- Encouraging a Growth Mindset: A growth mindset is the belief that abilities and intelligence can be developed through dedication and hard work. Leaders should encourage this mindset within their teams by celebrating progress, acknowledging effort, and promoting the idea that mistakes are opportunities to learn and grow.

PSYCHOLOGICAL SAFETY AND EMPOWERMENT

Psychological safety is the belief that one will not be penalized or humiliated for speaking up with ideas, questions, concerns, or mistakes. It is a critical factor in high-performing teams, especially in healthcare, where open communication and collaboration are essential for patient safety and team effectiveness. Leaders must create an environment where team members feel safe to express themselves, ask questions, challenge the status quo, and take risks without fear of negative consequences.

Building Psychological Safety

- Encouraging Open Communication: Leaders must create a culture where team members feel comfortable sharing their thoughts and concerns. This involves actively listening to their input, offering constructive feedback, and ensuring that all voices are heard. Leaders should model transparency by sharing information openly and making it clear that everyone's perspective is valued.

- Valuing Diverse Perspectives: A culture of psychological safety thrives when diverse perspectives are not only welcomed but actively encouraged. Leaders should create an environment where different ideas, backgrounds, and experiences are seen as assets. This approach fosters innovation, creativity, and improved decision-making.
- Supporting Risk-Taking: In healthcare, trying new approaches or speaking up about potential problems can be daunting, especially if team members fear criticism or retribution. Leaders must foster an environment where risk-taking is seen as an opportunity for growth and learning rather than something to be punished.
- Empowering Team Members: Empowerment goes hand-in-hand with psychological safety. Leaders should give team members the autonomy to make decisions, offer feedback, and take ownership of their work. When individuals feel empowered, they are more likely to be engaged, motivated, and contribute to the team's success.

DISCUSSION QUESTIONS

How can respiratory care leaders create a culture of psychological safety while maintaining high standards of patient care and professional accountability?

MODULE SIXTEEN

FUTURE-PROOF LEADERSHIP: PREPARING LEADERS AND DEPARTMENTS FOR GROWTH AND SUSTAINABILITY

In the dynamic and ever-evolving healthcare landscape, particularly in respiratory care, leadership must adapt and prepare for the future. Future-proof leadership ensures that organizations and departments are resilient, adaptable, and capable of thriving even in times of crisis and change. As healthcare systems continue to evolve, it is critical that leaders focus on building a sustainable foundation that will foster long-term growth, innovation, and stability.

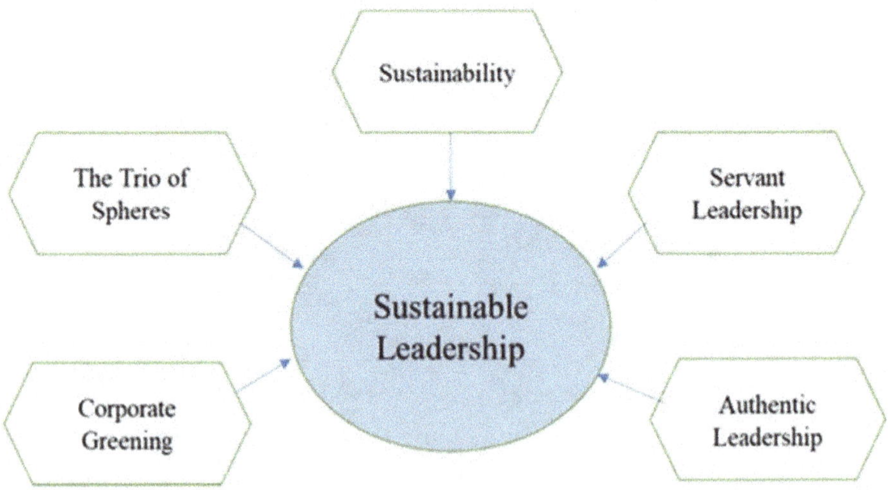

This section will explore the key aspects of future-proof leadership in respiratory care: Leading Through Crisis and Change, Creating Resilient and Agile Departments, Succession Planning and Leadership Development Programs, and Leaving a Lasting Legacy. These principles will enable respiratory leaders to navigate complex challenges, create adaptable teams, ensure the continuity of effective leadership, and leave a meaningful impact on the field.

LEADING THROUGH CRISIS AND CHANGE

The ability to lead through crisis and change is one of the most crucial aspects of future-proof leadership. In healthcare, crises are inevitable, whether they are driven by a global pandemic, economic downturns, or technological disruptions. Respiratory care leaders must be prepared to respond effectively, maintain operations, and keep teams motivated and focused on delivering high-quality patient care.

Key Aspects of Leading Through Crisis and Change

Adaptability and Flexibility: During crises, the ability to quickly adapt and adjust strategies is vital. Respiratory leaders must be able to shift priorities, adjust workflows, and implement temporary measures that ensure continuity of care. For instance, during the COVID-19 pandemic, respiratory care teams had to quickly adapt to new safety protocols, expand the use of ventilators, and manage an influx of patients in critical care.

- Clear Communication: Effective communication is critical during times of crisis. Leaders must keep their teams informed, provide transparent updates, and ensure that everyone is on the same page. Miscommunication during a crisis can lead to confusion, mistakes, and decreased morale. Respiratory leaders should use clear, concise language and provide regular updates about evolving circumstances, safety guidelines, and organizational priorities.
- Decision-Making Under Pressure: Leading through crisis requires strong decision-making skills. Respiratory leaders often need to make tough decisions quickly, balancing short-term needs with long-term goals. In a crisis, these decisions might involve resource allocation (e.g., ventilator distribution), staff reorganization, or adjustments to patient care protocols. Respiratory leaders should be prepared to make data-driven, evidence-based decisions that prioritize patient safety and care quality.
- Emotional Support for Teams: During periods of uncertainty, staff can experience high levels of stress, burnout, and anxiety. Respiratory leaders should provide emotional support for their teams, acknowledging their

concerns, offering encouragement, and creating opportunities for mental health support. Leaders should foster an environment where staff feel comfortable discussing their challenges and seeking assistance.

- Resilience in Leadership: Leaders must demonstrate resilience by maintaining composure, showing empathy, and setting a positive example. Resilient leaders inspire confidence in their teams, showing that they are capable of navigating difficult situations. By exhibiting calmness and focus, respiratory leaders can help their teams stay grounded and stay on track.
- Innovation in Response to Crisis: Crises often spur innovation. Respiratory care leaders should embrace new technologies, workflows, and treatment strategies that emerge during crises. For example, during the COVID-19 pandemic, telemedicine and remote monitoring became essential tools for providing care to respiratory patients while minimizing exposure to healthcare workers.

CREATING RESILIENT AND AGILE DEPARTMENTS

Resilience and agility are essential qualities for any department aiming for long-term success. In respiratory care, departments must be prepared for unexpected changes in patient demand, resource availability, or external circumstances. Building resilience and agility within respiratory departments ensures that they can continue to provide high-quality care, even in the face of adversity.

Key Principles of Resilient and Agile Departments

Fostering a Growth Mindset: Resilient and agile departments have a culture of continuous learning and improvement. Respiratory care leaders should encourage their teams to embrace a growth mindset, where challenges are seen as opportunities for development. This mindset helps teams to remain adaptable, learn from setbacks, and grow stronger in the process.

- Cross-Training and Skill Diversification: One of the key strategies for creating agile departments is cross-training staff. Cross-training ensures that team members have a variety of skills and can step into different roles when needed. In respiratory care, this might involve training therapists to perform both inpatient and outpatient care or preparing staff to work in both critical care and routine pulmonary rehabilitation settings. Cross-training increases the department's flexibility and enables staff to respond to changing needs more effectively.

- Resource Management and Optimization: To remain resilient, respiratory departments need to optimize their resources, both human and material. Leaders should regularly assess staff workloads, equipment usage, and supply chain needs to ensure that resources are available and allocated efficiently. For example, during times of high demand, such as flu season or a respiratory virus outbreak, departments should ensure that equipment like ventilators and oxygen supplies are stocked and ready for use.
- Scenario Planning and Preparedness: Scenario planning helps departments anticipate potential challenges and develop strategies to address them. Respiratory leaders should engage in regular risk assessments and planning exercises to prepare for various contingencies, such as spikes in patient volume, staffing shortages, or supply chain disruptions. These plans should include protocols for quickly mobilizing resources, adjusting staffing levels, and ensuring patient care continuity.
- Support for Work-Life Balance: A resilient department must support the well-being of its staff. Respiratory care leaders should create a work environment that allows employees to manage work-life balance effectively. This can be achieved by offering flexible scheduling, mental

health support, and wellness initiatives. Resilient employees are more likely to stay engaged and motivated, even during challenging times.

- Encouraging Innovation and Flexibility: Agility requires the ability to innovate and quickly implement new solutions. Respiratory leaders should encourage staff to share ideas for process improvements, new technologies, and novel approaches to patient care. Flexibility in adapting these innovations is key to ensuring the department can pivot quickly when needed.

SUCCESSION PLANNING AND LEADERSHIP DEVELOPMENT PROGRAMS

Succession planning is essential to ensure that an organization's leadership pipeline remains strong and that departments are prepared for future changes. In respiratory care, where skilled professionals are in high demand, creating a leadership development program ensures that the department has a steady supply of competent leaders who can take on critical roles in the future.

Building Effective Succession Planning

Identifying Key Leadership Roles: The first step in succession planning is to identify key leadership roles within the department, including department heads, team leads, and specialized leadership positions. These roles are essential for ensuring the department's success and continuity, and it is important to have potential successors ready to step in as needed.

- Talent Identification and Development: Respiratory leaders should actively identify potential leaders within their teams. This involves recognizing employees who demonstrate leadership potential, such as strong communication skills, problem-solving abilities, and a deep understanding of clinical practices. Once identified, these individuals should be provided with the necessary training, mentoring, and development opportunities to prepare them for leadership roles.
- Mentoring and Coaching Programs: Mentoring and coaching are crucial components of leadership development. Senior respiratory leaders should actively mentor and guide emerging leaders, helping them navigate the challenges of leadership roles and providing support as they gain experience. This can include one-on-one coaching, leadership training seminars, and opportunities to lead small projects or teams.
- Encouraging Diverse Leadership: To create a truly effective leadership pipeline, respiratory departments should encourage diversity in leadership. This includes fostering an environment where individuals from

different backgrounds, experiences, and perspectives are given the opportunity to lead. Diversity in leadership leads to more innovative problem-solving and a better understanding of the needs of diverse patient populations.

- Preparing for Change: Succession planning also involves preparing for organizational changes. This can include anticipating retirements, role shifts, and changes in the healthcare landscape. Respiratory care leaders should be proactive in developing a pool of skilled candidates ready to step into leadership positions when the need arises.

YOUR LEGACY: LEAVING A LASTING IMPACT

As respiratory care leaders, it is important to consider the legacy they will leave behind. A legacy is not just about personal achievements, but about the impact made on the team, the patients, and the broader healthcare community. Leaders in respiratory care have the opportunity to influence the practice, mentor future leaders, and establish a culture of excellence that endures beyond their tenure.

Creating a Lasting Legacy

Mentorship and Knowledge Transfer: One of the most powerful ways to leave a lasting legacy is through mentorship. Respiratory care leaders who take the time to invest in the growth and development of their staff will ensure that their knowledge and values are passed down to future generations of professionals. This not only improves the department’s performance but also helps shape the future of the profession.

- Establishing a Culture of Excellence: Leaders can create a lasting impact by fostering a culture of excellence that prioritizes patient care, continuous learning, and collaboration. This culture will continue to influence the organization long after the leader has moved on, ensuring that the values they instilled remain central to the department's operations.
- Driving Innovation and Change: Leaders who champion innovation and process improvement leave behind a legacy of progress. By embracing new technologies, treatment methods, and ways of working, respiratory leaders can shape the future of care delivery and ensure that their department remains on the cutting edge.
- Advocacy for the Profession: Leaving a lasting legacy also involves advocating for the respiratory care profession on a larger scale. Leaders can promote the importance of respiratory care in the healthcare system, push for increased funding, and champion policies that benefit patients and professionals alike. By advocating for the profession, leaders help to elevate its status and ensure its future success.

- Inspiring Others to Lead: Finally, a strong legacy is built on inspiring others to lead. Respiratory care leaders who lead with integrity, compassion, and innovation set an example for others to follow. By encouraging others to step into leadership roles, leaders ensure that the profession will continue to thrive and evolve for years to come.

DISCUSSION QUESTIONS

- How can respiratory care leaders build a resilient and agile department that is able to thrive during times of change and crisis?
- What are the key elements of an effective leadership development program, and how can these be integrated into succession planning for respiratory care departments?

CONCLUSION

Leadership is an act intentional, bold, and compassionate that begins with a decision to serve others while holding yourself to the highest standard of care.

In respiratory therapy, every breath matters. And so does every decision, every interaction, every effort to uplift a colleague, advocate for a patient, or challenge the status quo. The kind of leadership that transforms departments, inspires teams, and improves lives is built day by day through consistency, empathy, accountability, and vision.

Throughout this book, we've explored the multifaceted nature of leadership in respiratory care. You've learned about team culture, communication, conflict resolution, innovation, succession planning, and the practical tools that support growth and sustainability. You've seen how to develop others, elevate your department, and drive measurable clinical excellence while never losing sight of the people behind the procedures.

But more than anything, this journey has asked you to look inward.

True leadership begins with self-awareness. It grows through service. It strengthens through resilience. And it lives on in those you've mentored, empowered, and inspired. As you take what you've learned and step forward whether into a new role or a renewed sense of purpose remember that your influence doesn't end when the shift does. You are building a legacy every single day.

The challenges in healthcare will never disappear. But the world needs leaders who run toward challenge with hope, who choose collaboration over competition, and who breathe life into teams by building cultures of trust, growth, and excellence. You are that leader.

So carry this knowledge forward. Share it. Live it. Teach it. Use your voice. Shape your team. And lead in a way that leaves no doubt: respiratory care is not just a specialty, it's a calling and your leadership is essential.

REFERENCES

- Alvesson, M., & Sveningsson, S. (2015). *Changing organizational culture: Cultural change work in progress*
- Baker, G. R., & Denis, J. L. (2011). *Medical leadership in health care systems: From professional authority to organizational leadership. Public Money & Management.*
- Barker, P., & Buchanan-Barker, P. (2011). *The tidal model: A guide for mental health professionals. Routledge.*
- Berwick, D. M., Nolan, T. W., & Whittington, J. (2008). *The Triple Aim: Care, health, and cost.*
- Bleich, M. R., & Hessler, K. (2016). *Developing leadership skills in a changing healthcare environment. Health Administration Press.*
- Brookfield, S. D. (2017). *Becoming a critically reflective teacher (2nd ed.). Jossey-Bass.*
- Carter, L., Ulrich, D., & Goldsmith, M. (2005). *Best practices in leadership development and organization change. Pfeiffer.*

- Daly, J., Speedy, S., & Jackson, D. (2015). *Contexts of nursing: An introduction (4th ed.). Elsevier Health Sciences.*
- Fischer, S. A. (2016). *Transformational leadership in nursing: A concept analysis. Nursing Forum,*
- Fraser, S. W., & Greenhalgh, T. (2001*). Coping with complexity: Educating for capability.*
- Gawande, A. (2010). *The checklist manifesto: How to get things right. Metropolitan Books.*
- Greenleaf, R. K. (2002). *Servant leadership: A journey into the nature of legitimate power and greatness (25th Anniversary Ed.). Paulist Press.*
- Kalisch, B. J., & Lee, H. (2010). *The impact of teamwork on missed nursing care. Nursing Outlook.*
- Kanter, R. M. (2004). *Confidence: How winning and losing streaks begin and end. Crown Business.*
- Maslow, A. H. (1943). *A theory of human motivation. Psychological Review.*
- Sinek, S. (2009). Start with why: *How great leaders inspire everyone to take action. Portfolio.*
- Stone, D., Patton, B., & Heen, S. (2010). *Difficult conversations: How to discuss what matters most. Penguin Books.*

- Studer, Q. (2003). *Hardwiring excellence: Purpose, worthwhile work, making a difference. Fire Starter Publishing.*
- Tannenbaum, S. I., & Salas, E. (2020). *Teams that work: The seven drivers of team effectiveness. Oxford University Press.*

www.ingramcontent.com/pod-product-compliance
Lightning Source LLC
LaVergne TN
LVHW022042200926
848481LV00003B/756
* 9 7 9 8 3 4 9 3 7 4 6 7 8 *